Are You a Physician?

A Small Story About a Big Problem in Medicine Today

Wherever the art of medicine is loved, there is also a love of humanity.

- Hippocrates

Are You a Physician?

A Small Story About a Big Problem in Medicine Today

Izzy Sensible, MD

Newman Medical Enterprises, Inc.
NewmanMedicalEnterprises.com
Pembroke Pines, FL

Paperback ISBN: 978-0-9967508-1-3

First Edition
October 2018

Dedicated to all physicians who agree patients have the right to know who is making critical healthcare decisions for them.

Better to be slapped with the
truth than kissed with a lie.

- Russian Proverb

Dear Reader,

Many years ago, I read the book *Are You My Mother?* to my children. Recently, I read the same book to my grandson. The simple drawings inspired me to write this book to share an important message.

Most people are unaware of the changes happening in medicine in America these days. The numbers and types of non-physician medical providers have increased significantly since I graduated medical school many years ago. People need to know that the doctors taking care of them in hospitals and clinics may not be physicians and do not have the same education and training as physicians.

In almost half of the states in the US, laws have been passed to allow nurse practitioners to practice medicine without physician supervision. Nurse practitioners who pass their licensing exams can claim they are board certified, but board certification means something completely different for physicians - completion of three or more years of residency and fellowship. Then comes a rigorous board certification examination which must be retaken every ten years. Nurse practitioners can easily change their medical specialty, whereas physicians would need to complete an additional three or more years of full time residency or fellowship training and pass another board examination.

Despite the protests of nurse practitioners and physician assistants about being called mid-level providers and physician extenders, those titles clearly explain the original intent of these clinician positions. They were never meant to practice medicine independently like a physician, whose extensive education and training makes them uniquely qualified to diagnose and prescribe medical treatment.

I want everyone to know that I love nurses. Over the years, nurses have been my partners in caring for thousands of patients and I deeply respect their dedication to helping people. With the explosion of nurse practitioner degree program in recent years, including online and part-time programs, many amazing nurses have left their jobs to become nurse practitioners. The nursing shortage in the US is becoming critical and many hospitals cannot find enough nurses to cover their needs.

Please do not send me messages saying that you can't verify my medical license online and therefore won't believe anything I say in this book. Izzy Sensible is not my legal name. Physicians who have spoken about their concerns regarding the practice of medicine by non-physicians have been attacked on social media, in the press, and some have even lost their jobs. Even though I have recently retired from the practice of medicine, I have decided to use a pen name.
- Izzy Sensible MD, October 2018

For more information on the issues discussed in this book, please visit:

Physicians for Patient Protection (PhysiciansForPatientProtection.org) and Physicians For Patients (PhysiciansForPatients.org).

There is also information with references on my website AreYouaPhysician.com.

Truth will ultimately prevail
where there is pains to
bring it to light.

- George Washington

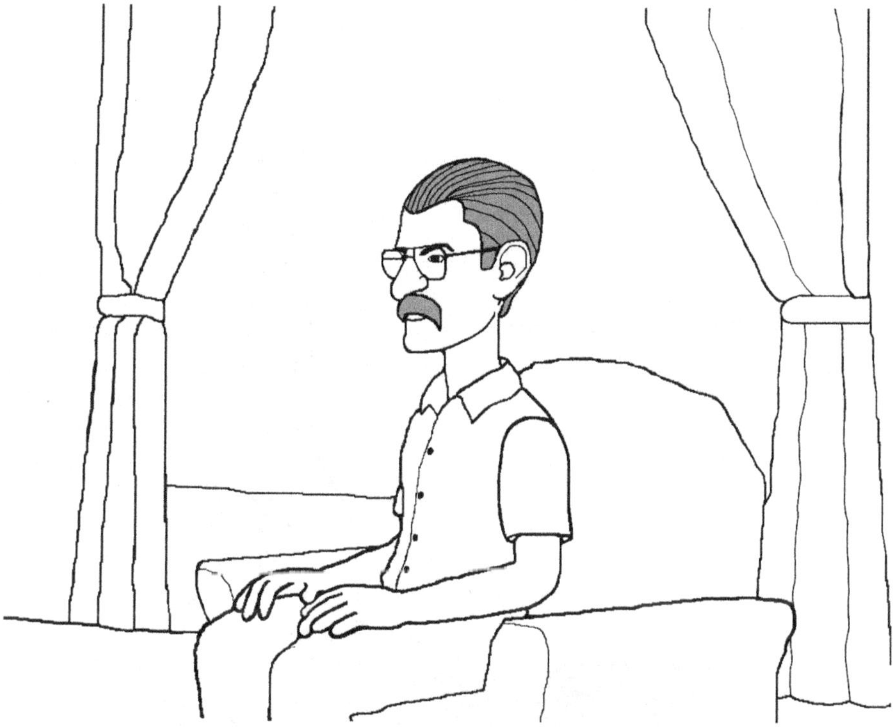

Dr. Smith was a retired family medicine physician. After his wife died, he lived alone.

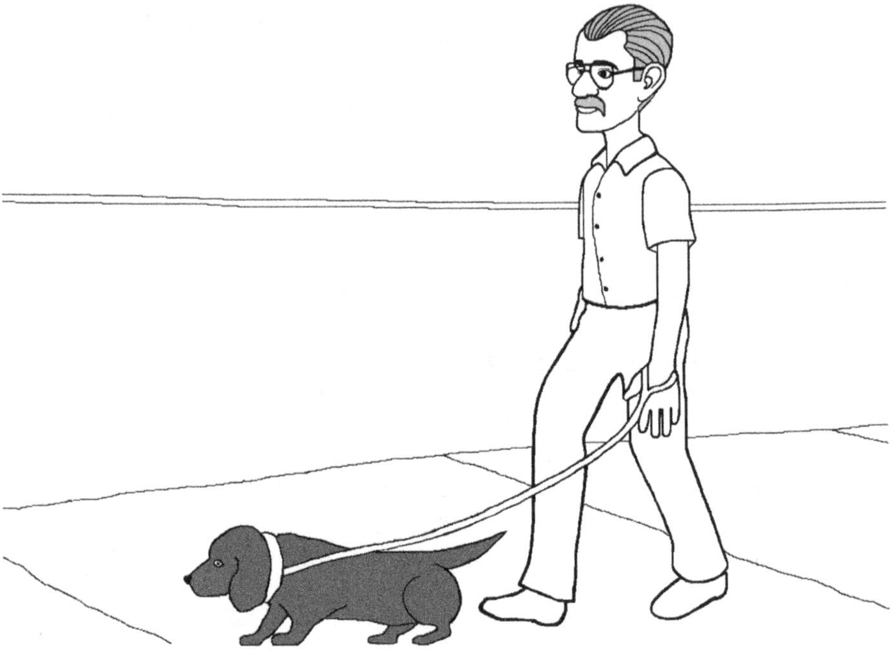

Every morning, Dr. Smith would go for a long walk with his dog in his retirement community.

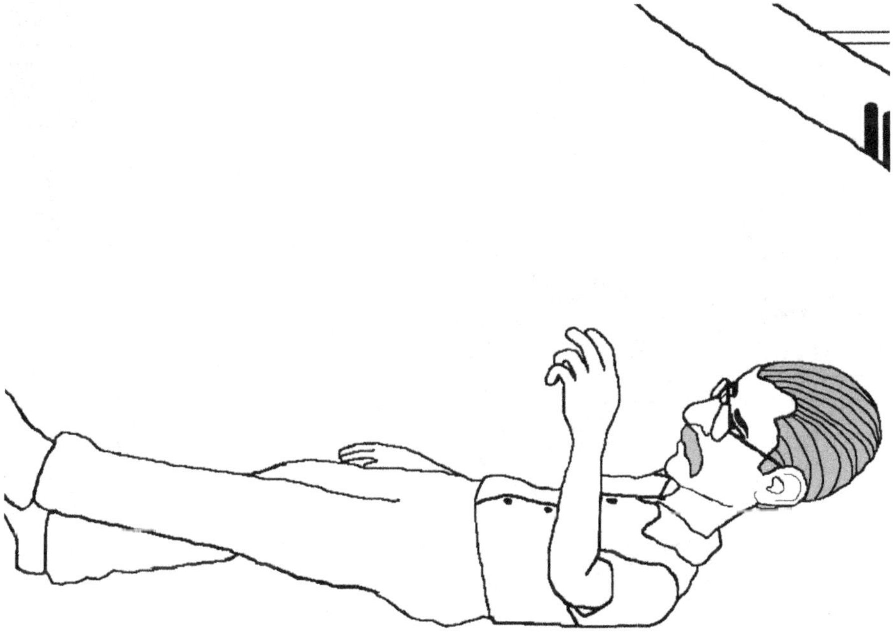

One morning, Dr. Smith tripped and fell while walking down the street. He knew his hip was broken when he could not stand up. A neighbor called for emergency help.

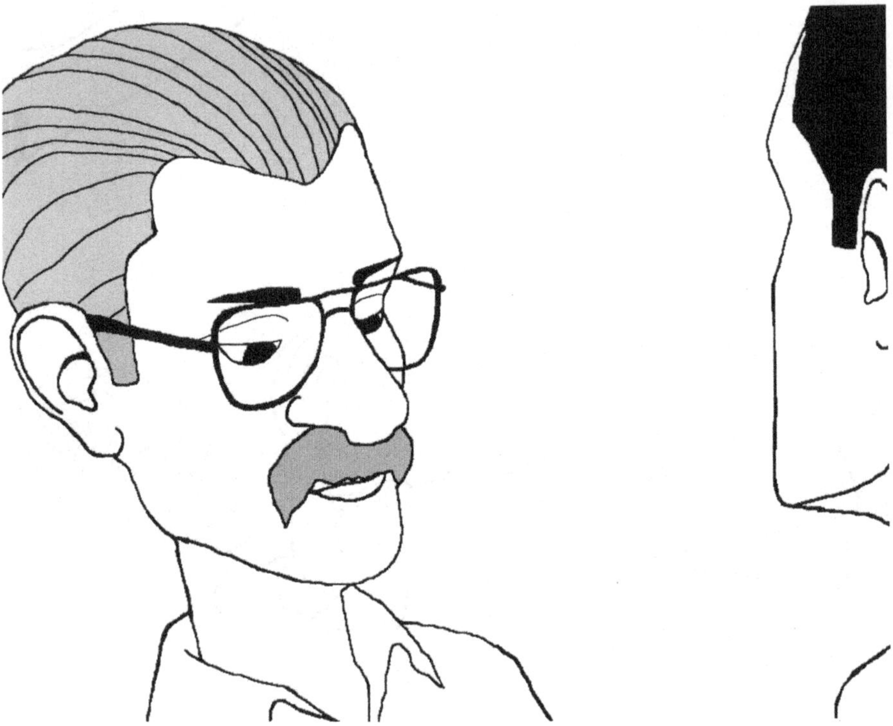

Dr. Smith noticed that the paramedic wore a name badge that said "Doc."

"Are you a physician?" asked Dr. Smith.

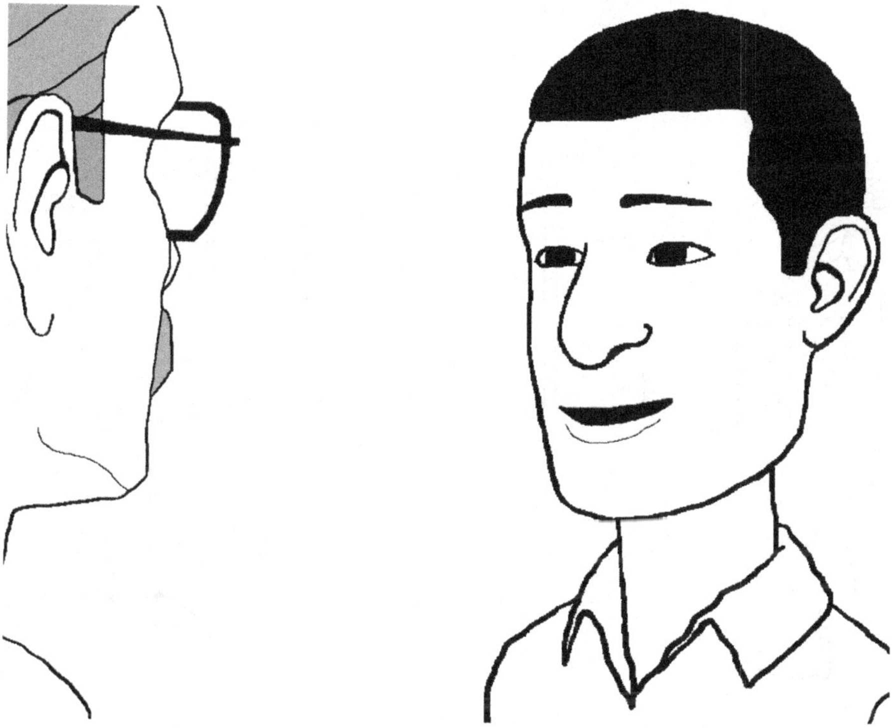

"No," answered the paramedic. "I have a PhD degree in philosophy, so the guys call me Doc."

Dr. Smith shook his head in disappointment.

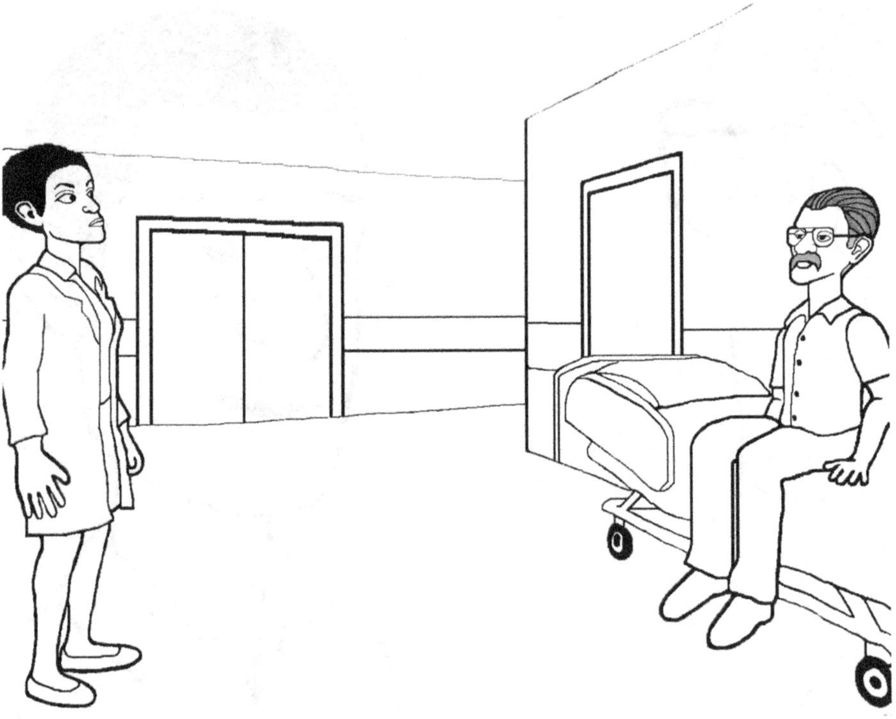

The ambulance arrived at the emergency room and Dr. Smith was taken inside. A woman wearing a white coat approached Dr. Smith and introduced herself as Dr. Rodriguez.

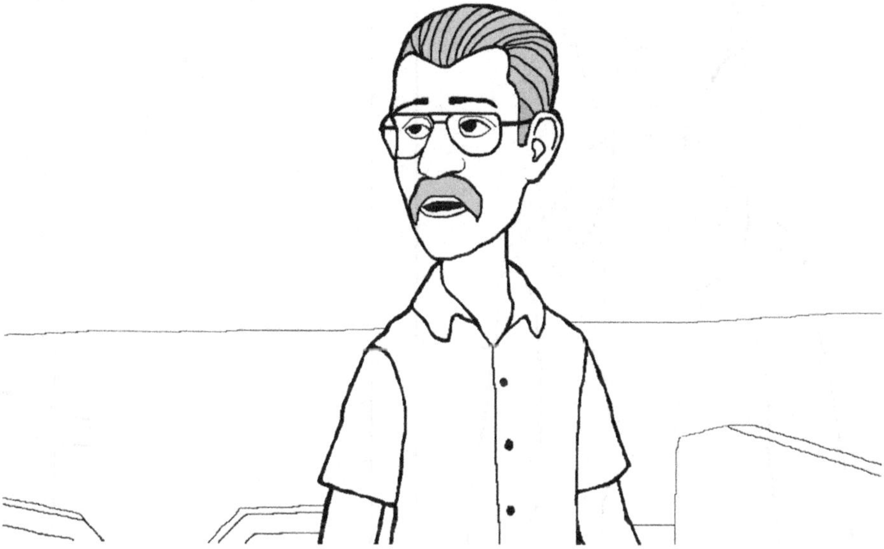

"Are you a physician?" asked Dr. Smith.

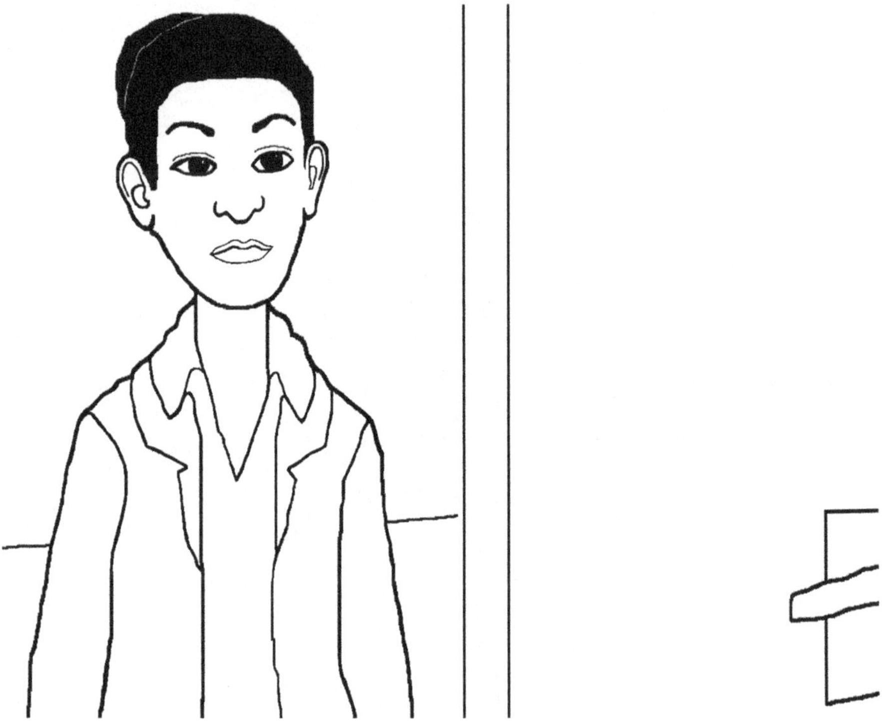

“No,” she replied. “I have a Doctorate of Nursing Practice, also known as a DNP degree. I am a nurse practitioner.”

Dr. Smith shook his head in disappointment.

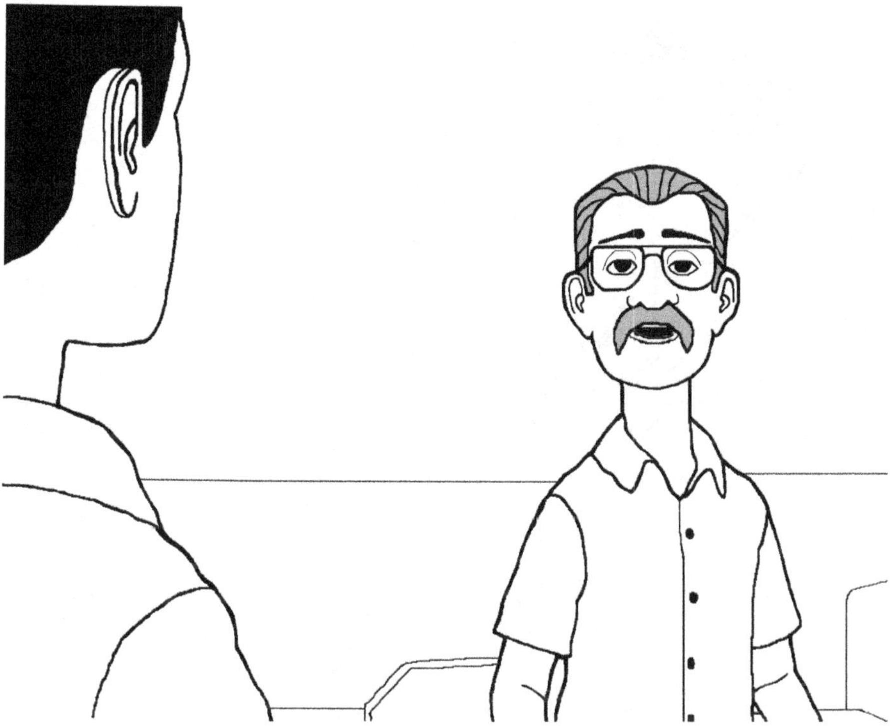

"How long were you a nurse before you went back to school?" asked Dr. Smith.

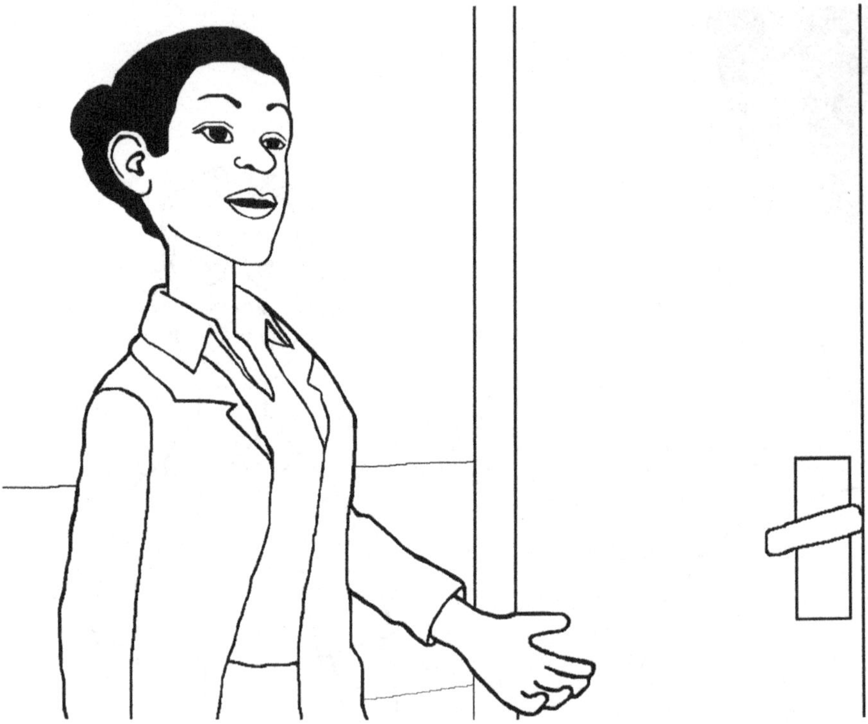

"I went straight from nursing school into a DNP program," she responded.

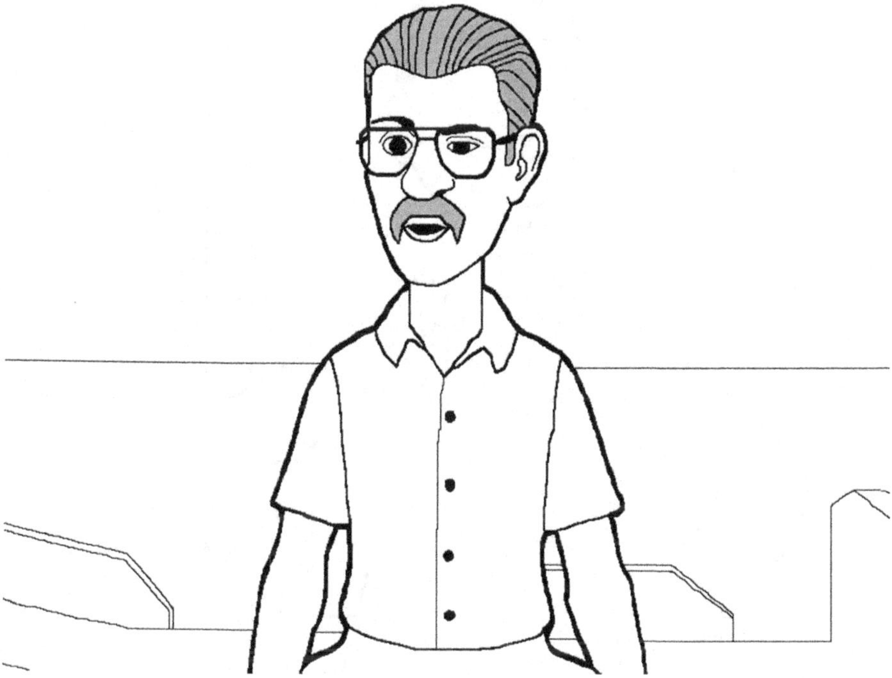

"How long was your training to become a nurse practitioner?" asked Dr. Smith.

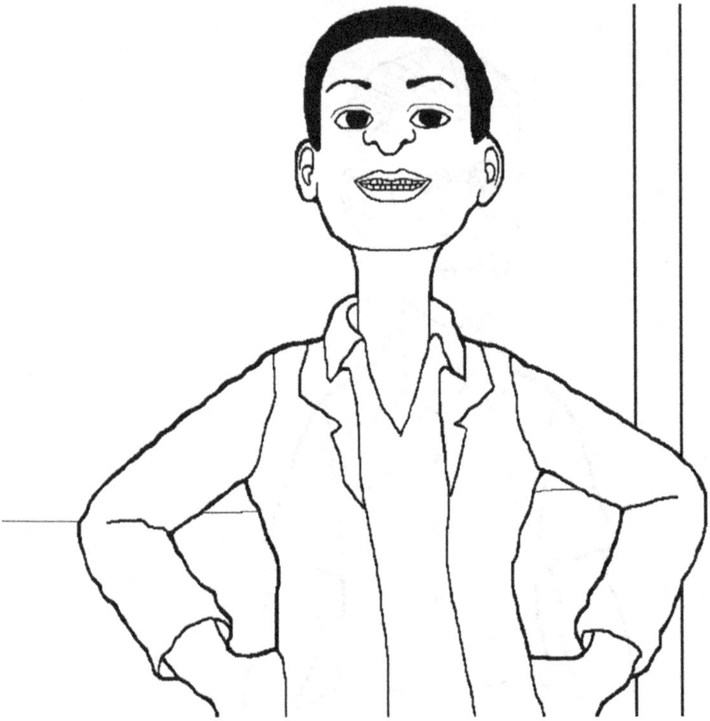

"It was a two year online program," the nurse practitioner answered, "and I was able to work full time while I did it."

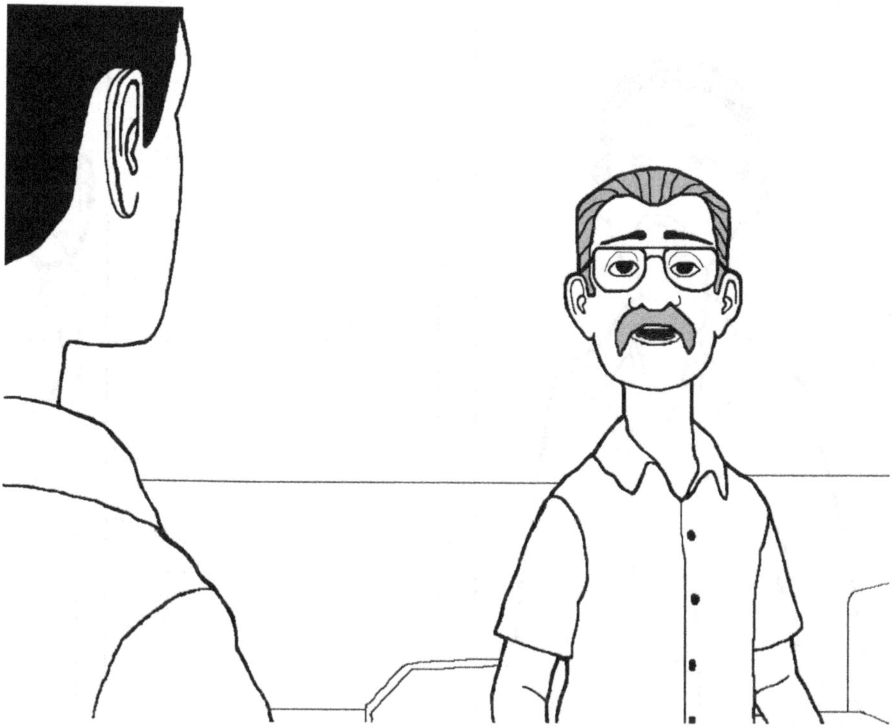

"How many hours of clinical training did you have to do?" asked Dr. Smith.

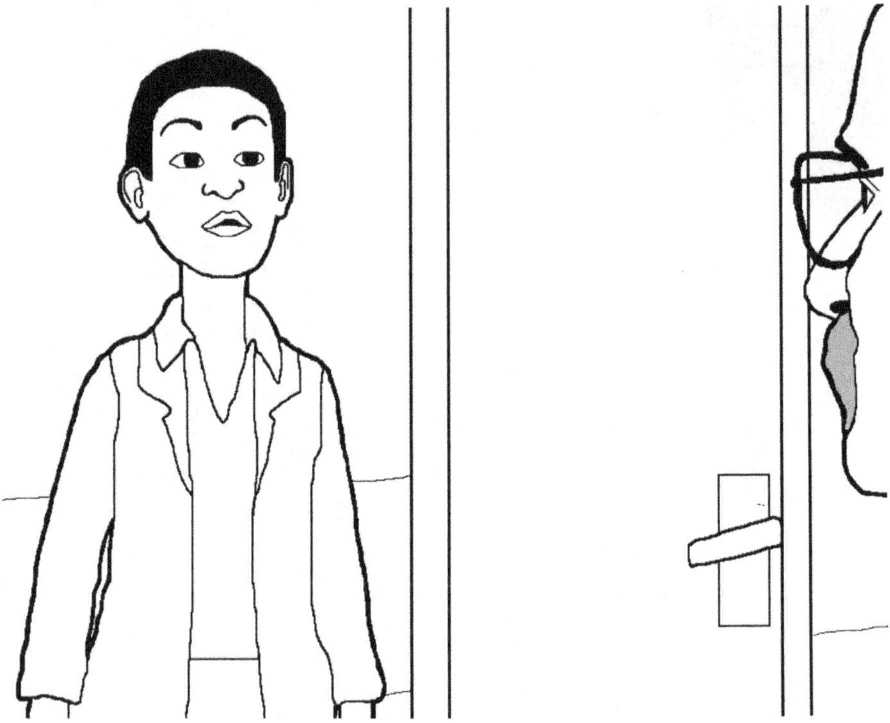

“Only 500 hours,” the nurse practitioner replied. “And it was mostly just following around other providers while they worked.”

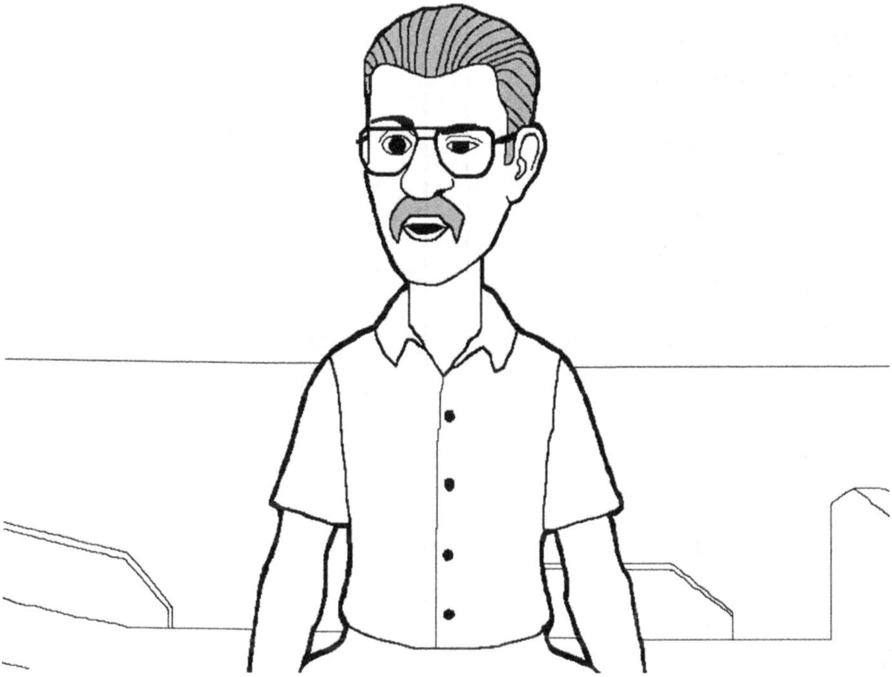

"When will I get to see the physician?" asked Dr. Smith.

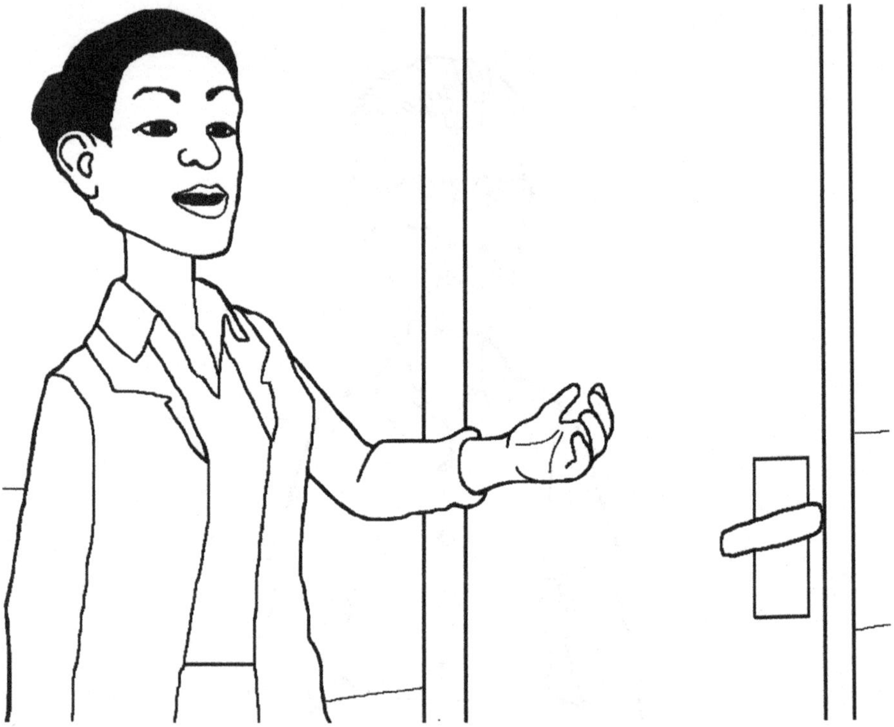

Our emergency room is staffed with only nurse practitioners," she replied.

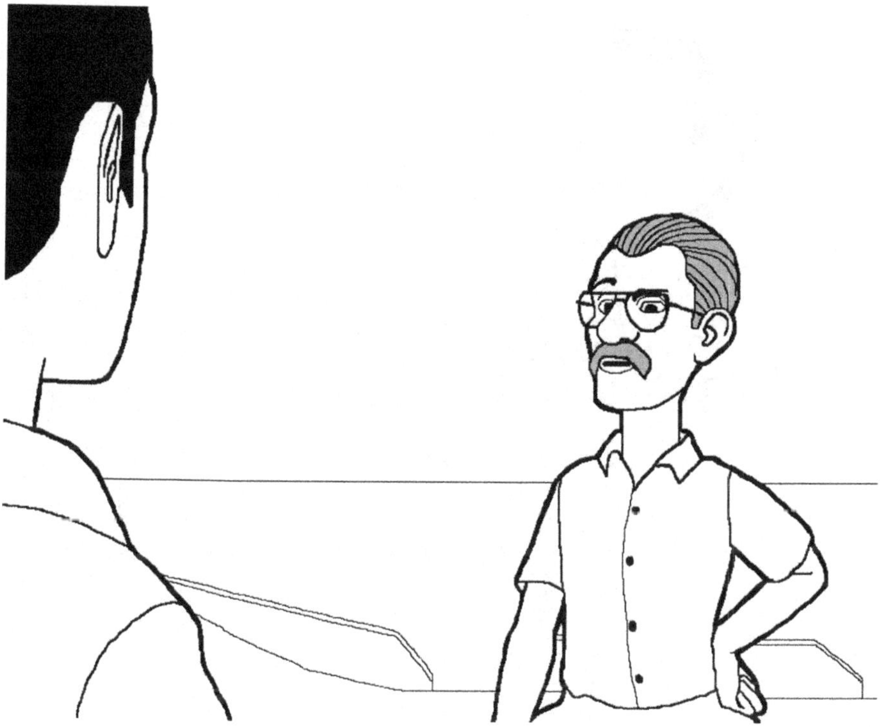

“But where is your supervising physician?” asked Dr. Smith.

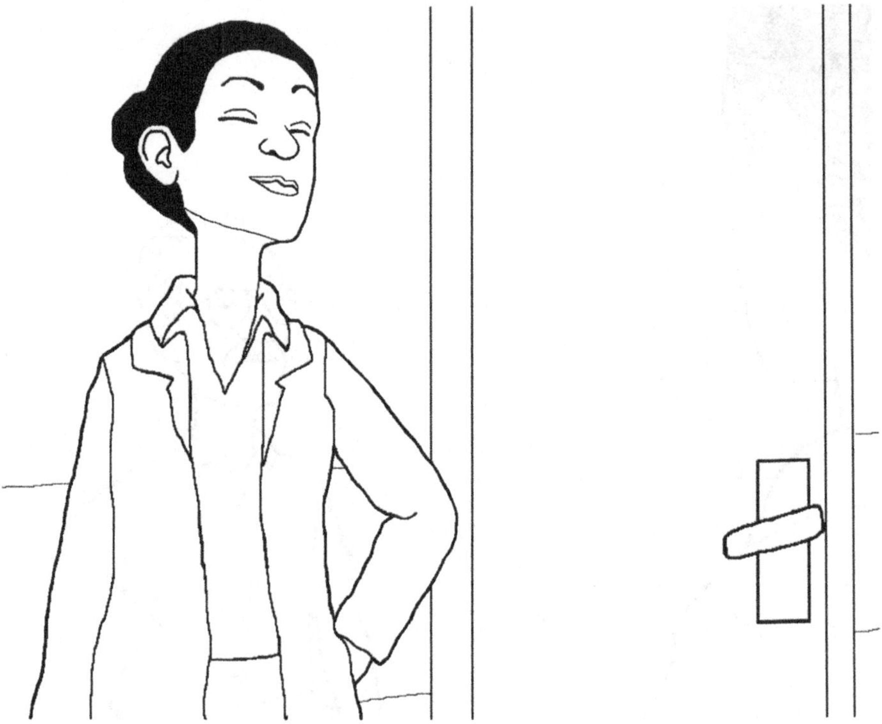

"Nurse practitioners now have full practice authority in this state. We no longer need a collaborating physician," she proudly responded.

"Nurse practitioners can do anything physicians can. We are even better than physicians because we spend more time with our patients."

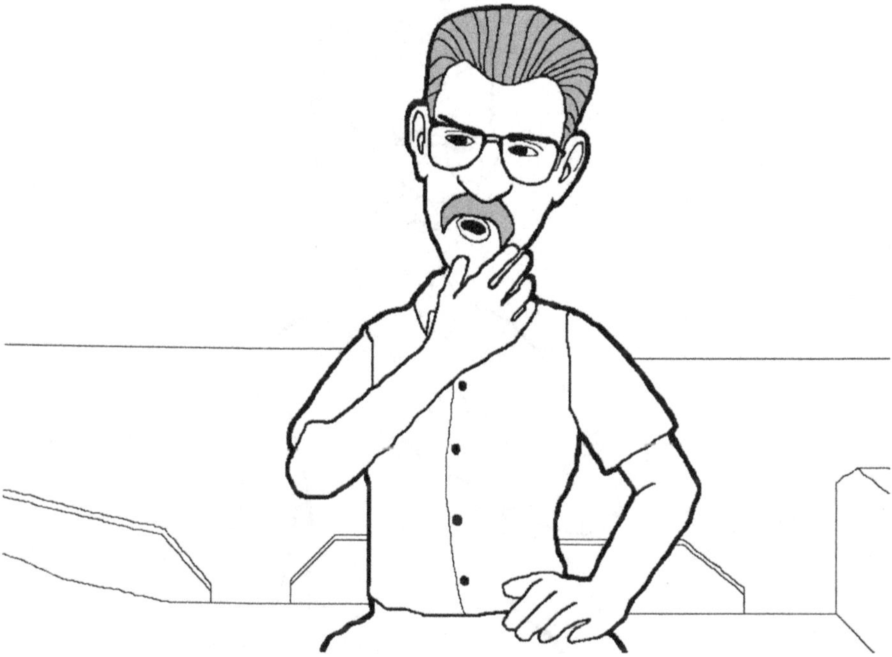

"But you didn't go to medical school," pointed out Dr. Smith. He quickly added up the numbers in his head. "And you only did about 3% of the over 15,000 hours of training I did during medical school and my three years of family medicine residency."

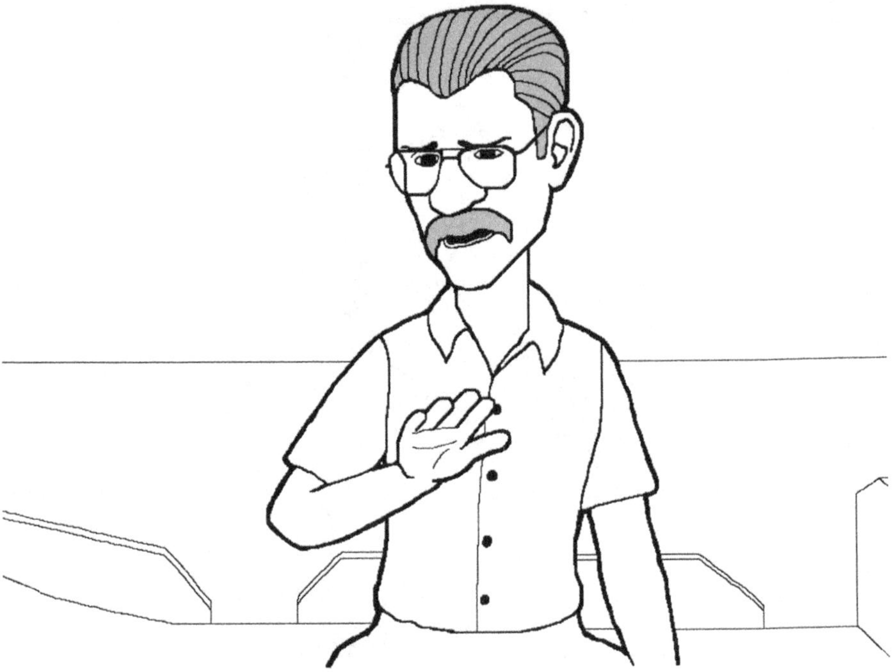

Dr. Smith was not happy. He refused to answer any more of the nurse practitioner's questions.

"Go away," Dr. Smith said and turned his face towards the wall. "I need a real doctor."

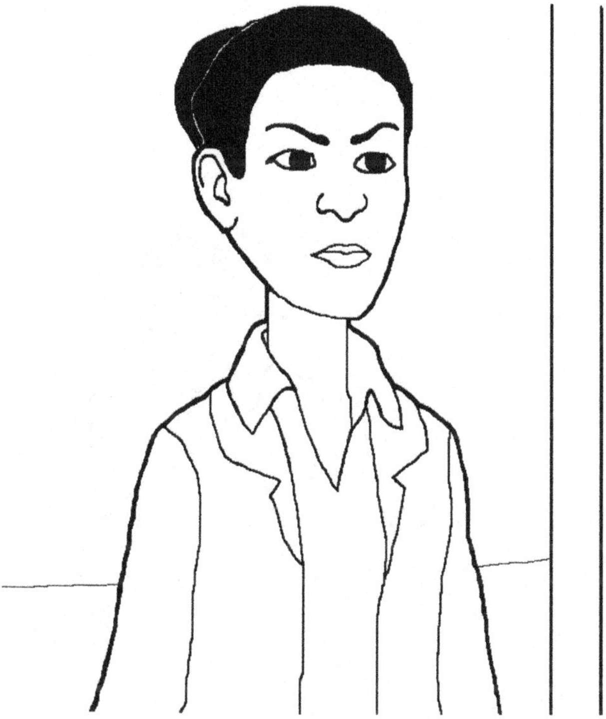

"I don't know why you are upset. Other patients don't complain about seeing a nurse practitioner instead of a physician." The nurse practitioner was surprised by Dr. Smith's reaction.

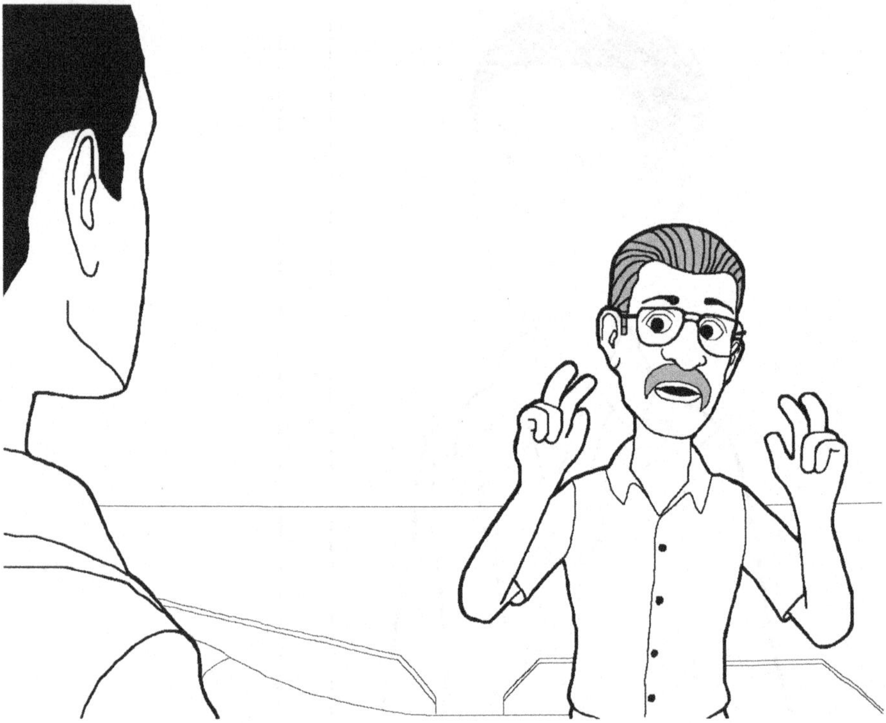

"That's because they don't know you are not a real doctor," said Dr. Smith. He made air quotes with his fingers and rolled his eyes.

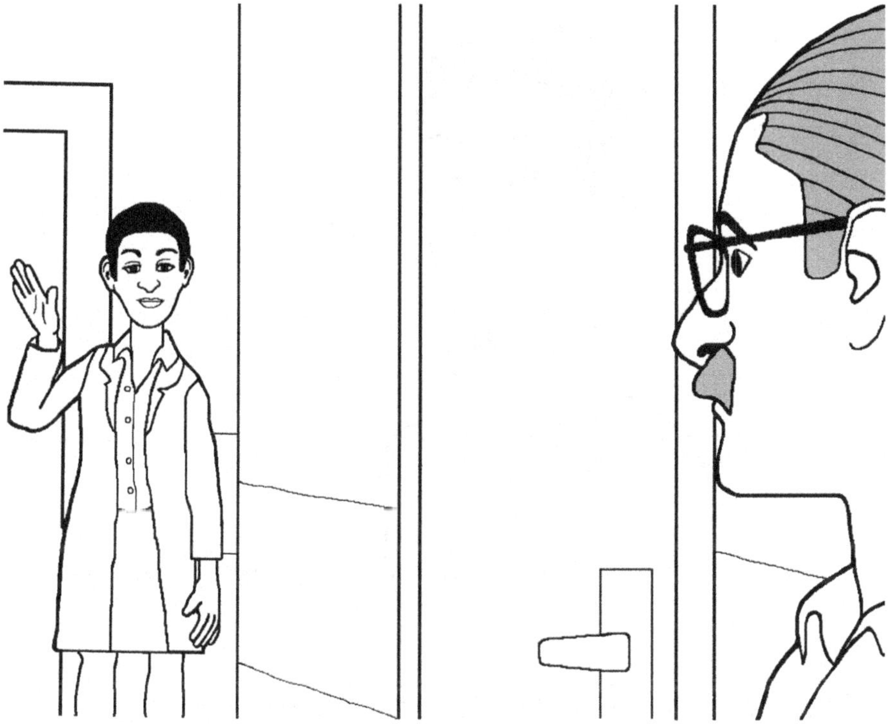

The nurse practitioner left the room and ordered x-rays of Dr. Smith's hip.

Dr. Smith was taken to get x-rays. After he was brought back to the emergency room, the nurse practitioner returned to see him.

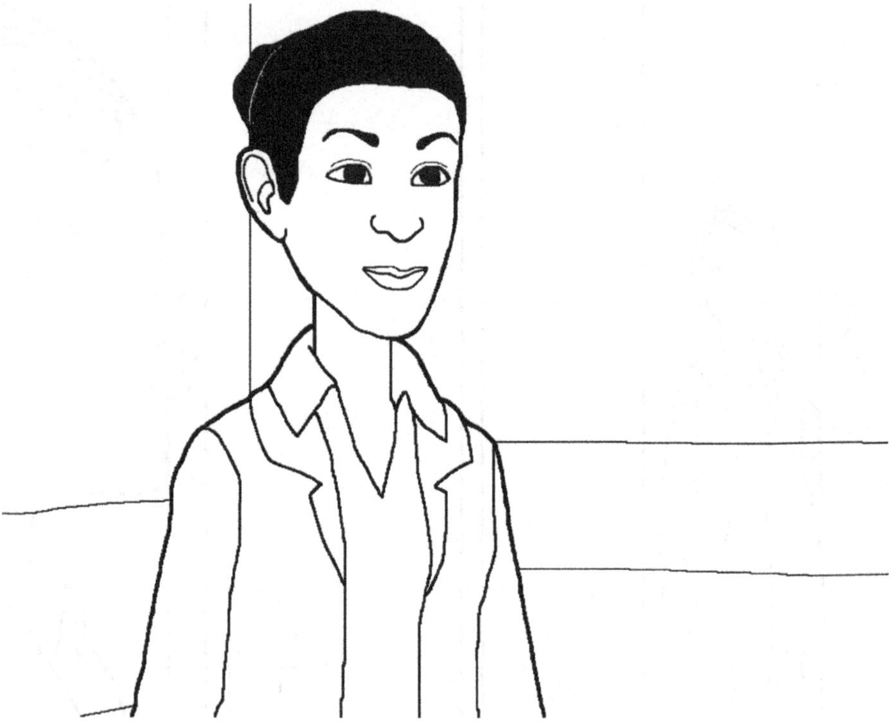

“You broke your hip,” said the nurse practitioner.

“What part?” asked Dr. Smith.

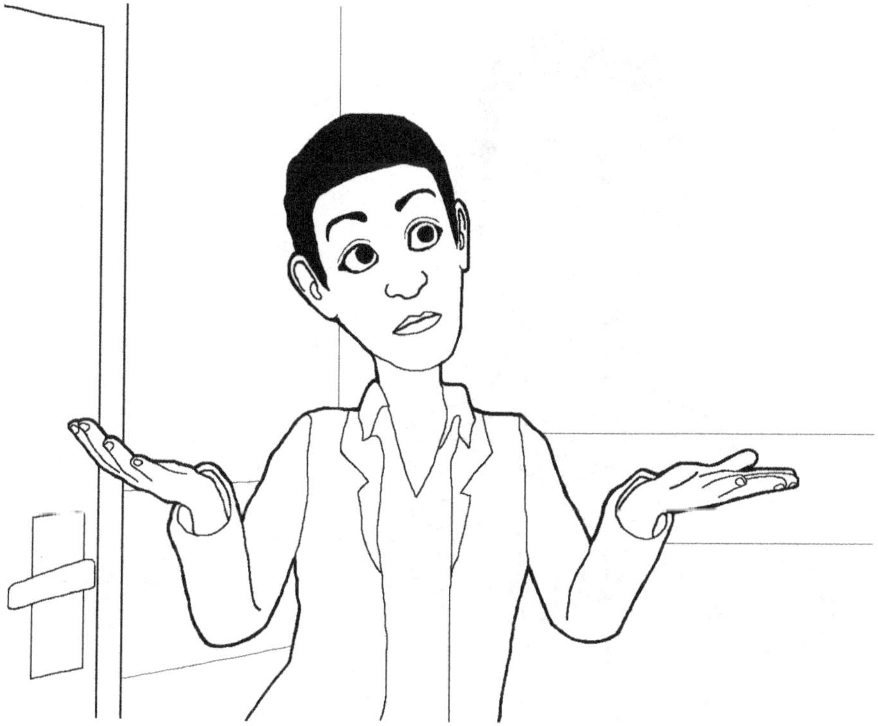

“I don’t know,” said the nurse practitioner.

“How bad is the fracture?” asked Dr. Smith.

“I don’t know,” said the nurse practitioner.

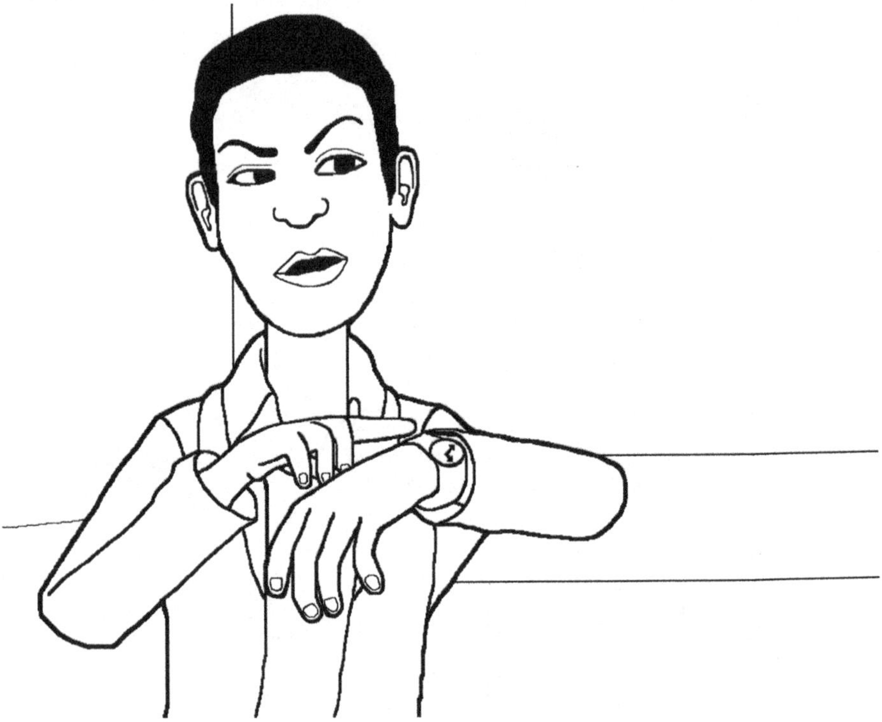

"The radiology technician only said it was broken," said the nurse practitioner. "The x-ray report is not back yet."

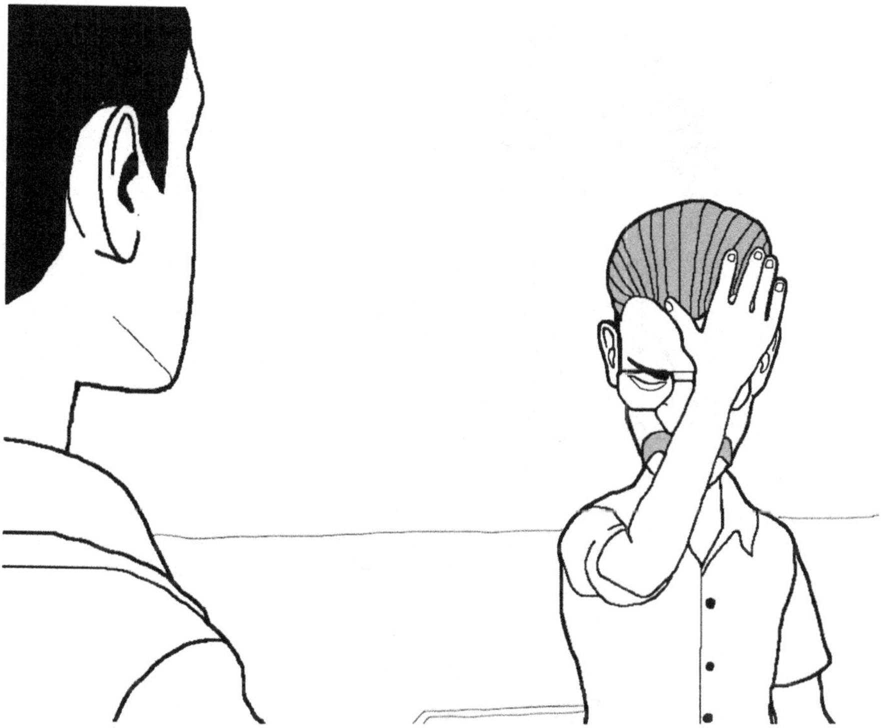

"You didn't look at the x-rays?" asked Dr. Smith. He was getting frustrated.

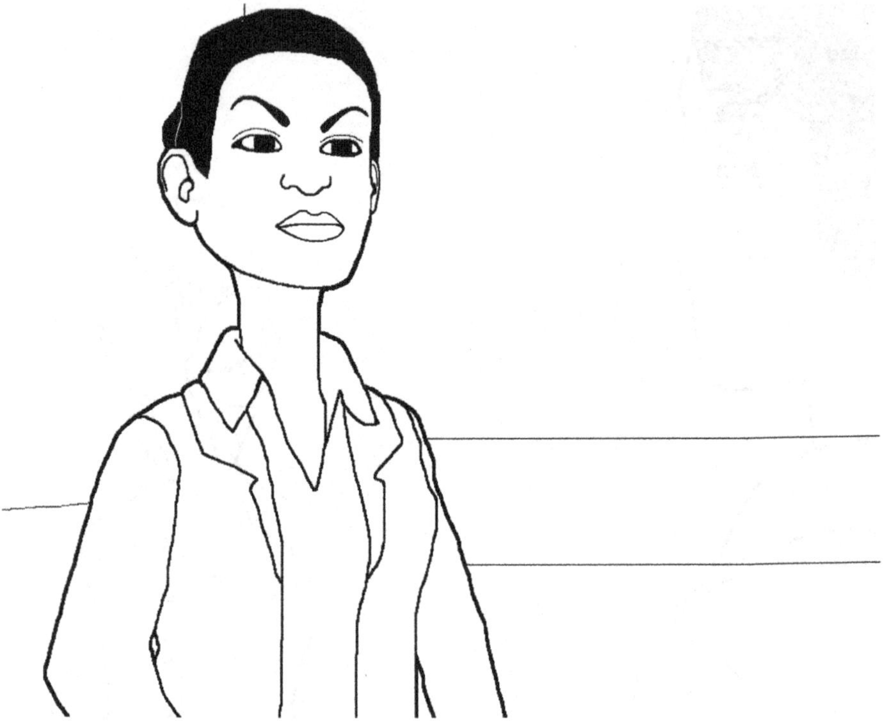

"I never do that," explained the nurse practitioner. "I just wait for the official report. Besides, reading x-rays wasn't part of my training."

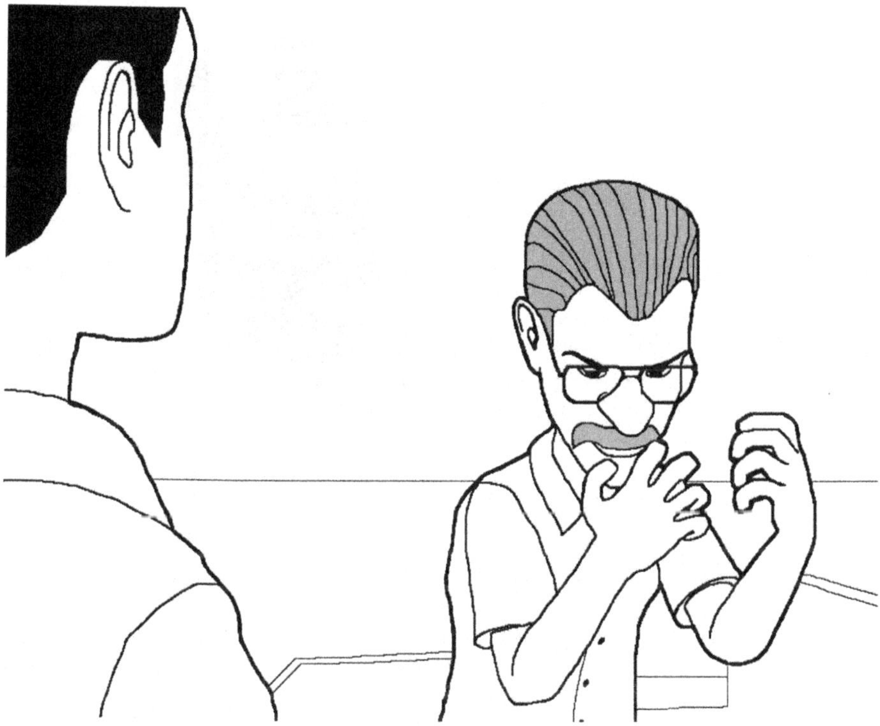

"Get out of my sight," shouted Dr. Smith. "I need a real doctor and an orthopedic surgeon."

Dr. Smith refused to answer any more of her questions so the nurse practitioner shrugged her shoulders and left.

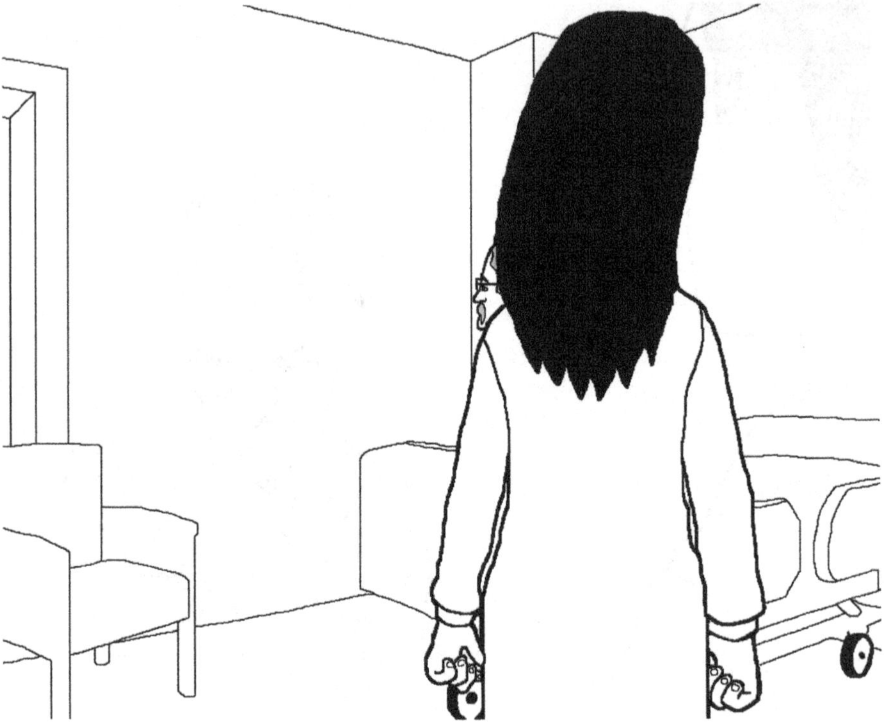

Dr. Smith was moved to a hospital room. A woman wearing a white coat entered the room and introduced herself as Dr. Abiaka.

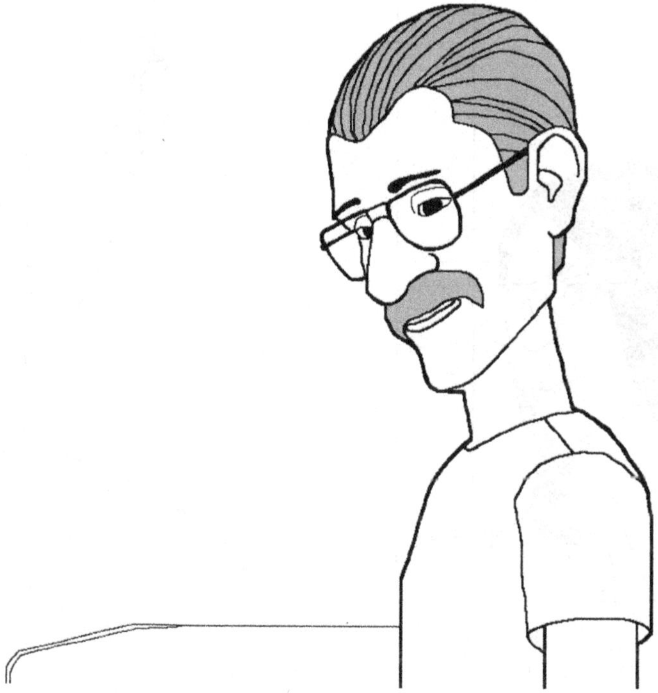

"Are you a physician?" asked Dr. Smith.

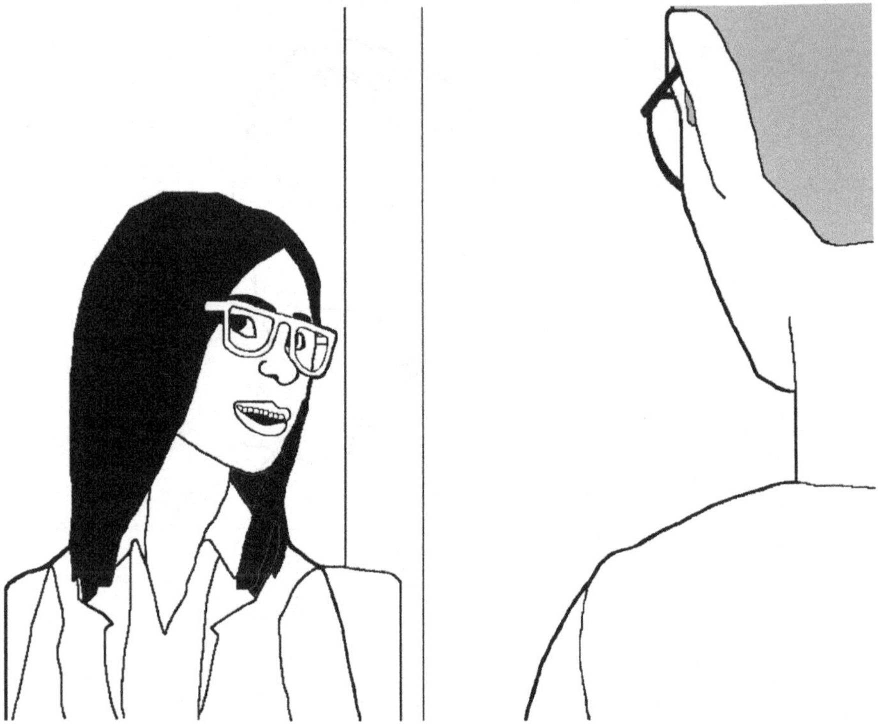

“No,” she replied. “I am a doctor of pharmacy with a PharmD degree. I need to review the list of your home medications.”

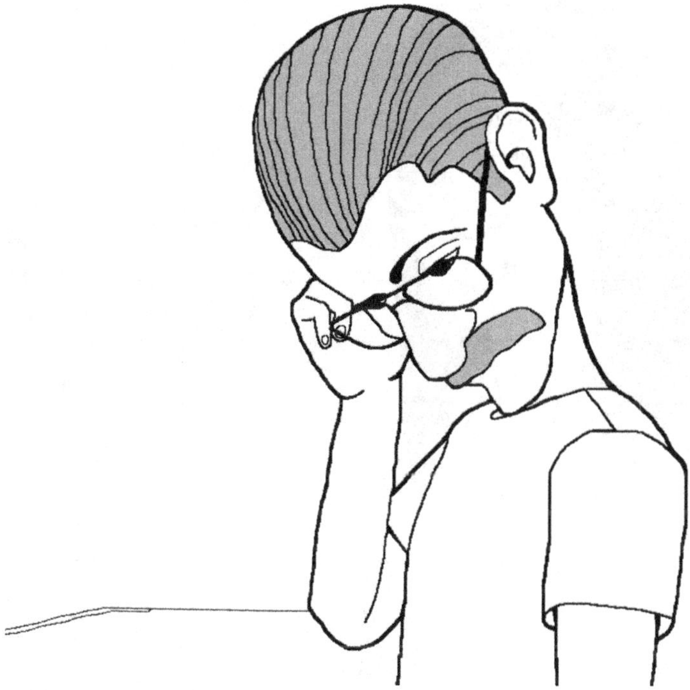

“Another doctor who is not a physician?” Dr Smith asked. “I gave them the list of my medications when I came to the hospital. Go away.”

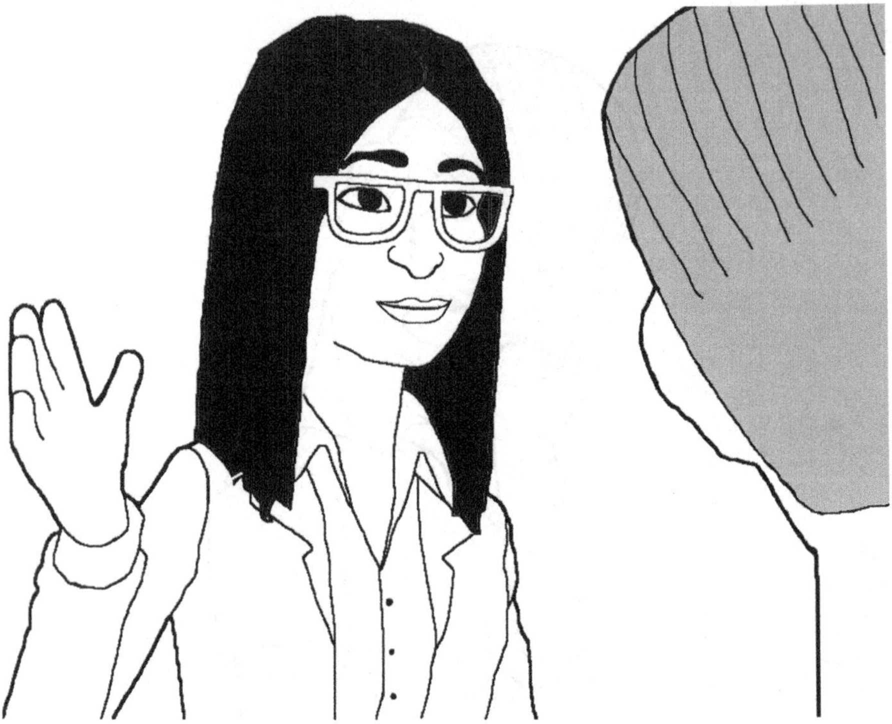

The pharmacist left Dr. Smith's room.

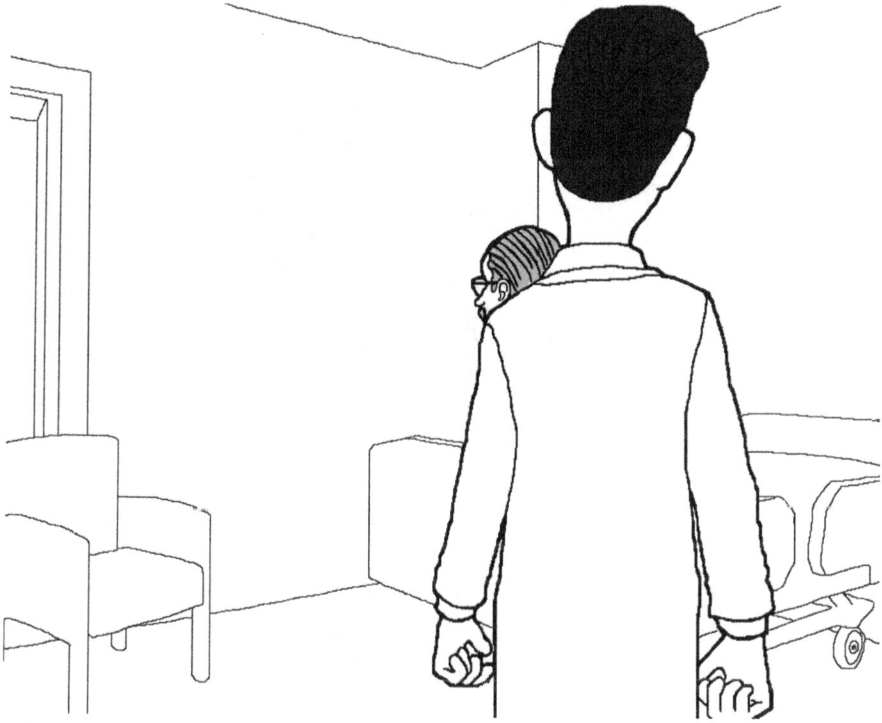

A man wearing a white coat entered the room and introduced himself as Dr. Jones.

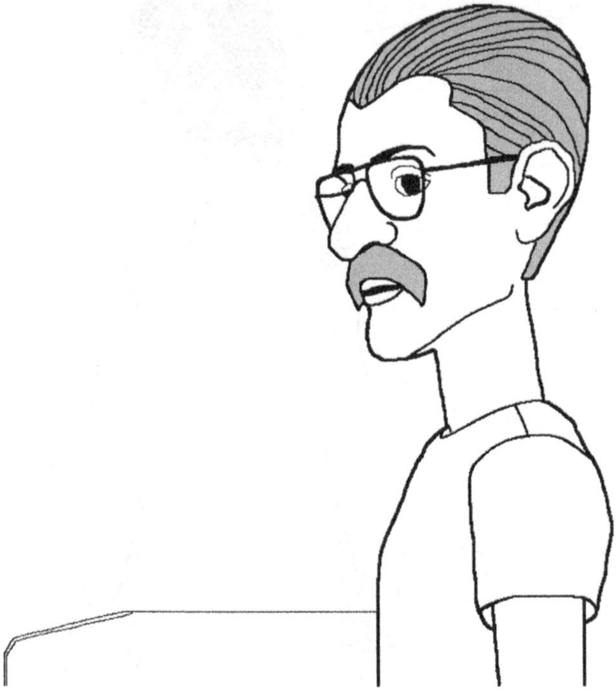

"Please have a seat. Are you a physician?" asked Dr. Smith.

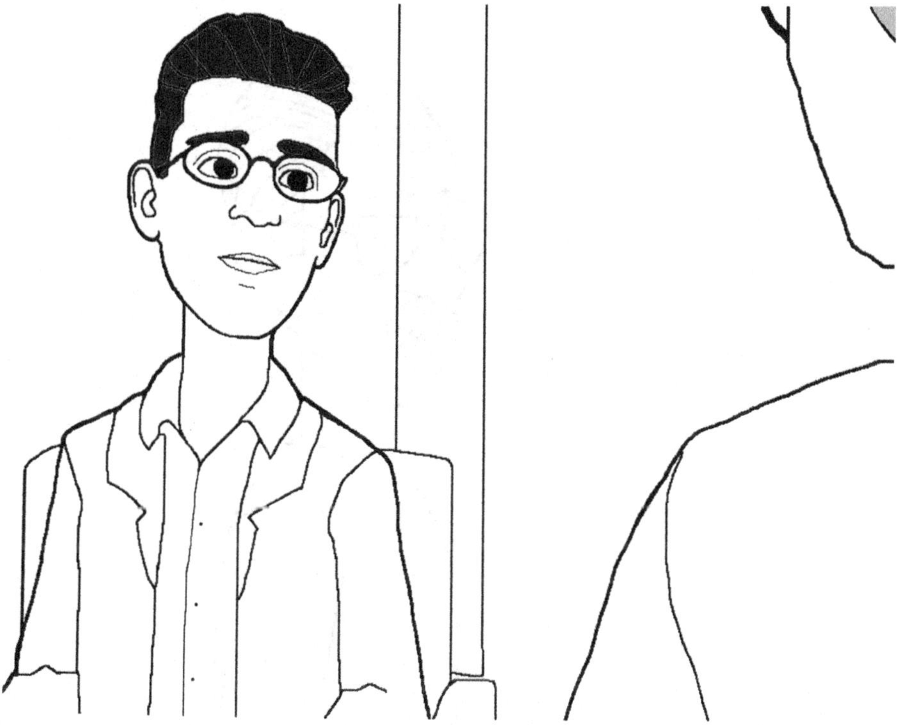

"No," he answered. "I am a physician associate."

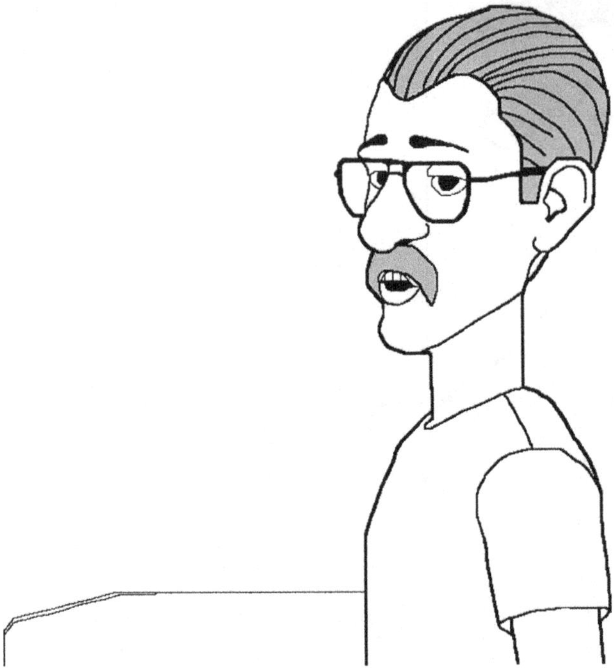

“What is that?” asked Dr. Smith. “I have never heard of that title before.”

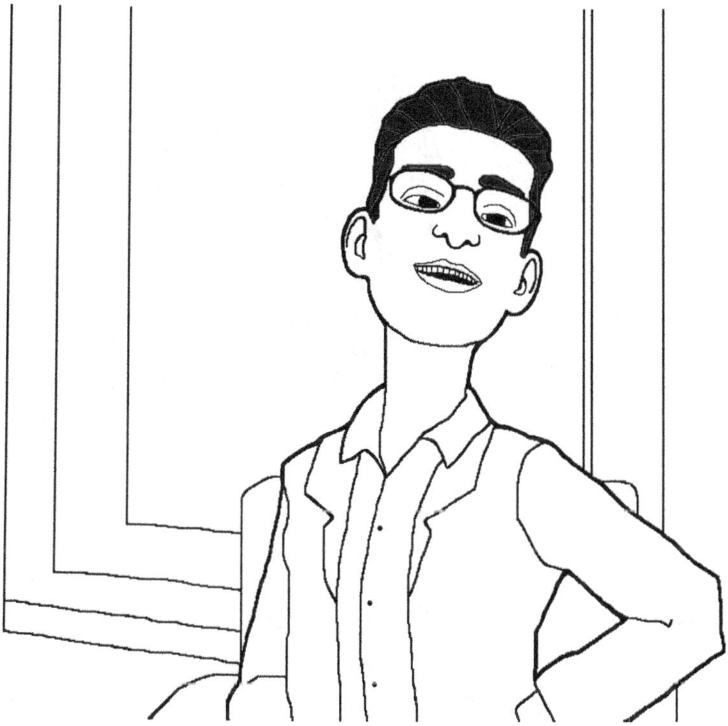

"We used to be called physician assistants. But that name implies that we cannot treat patients on our own. We think the title physician associate suits us better," he answered.

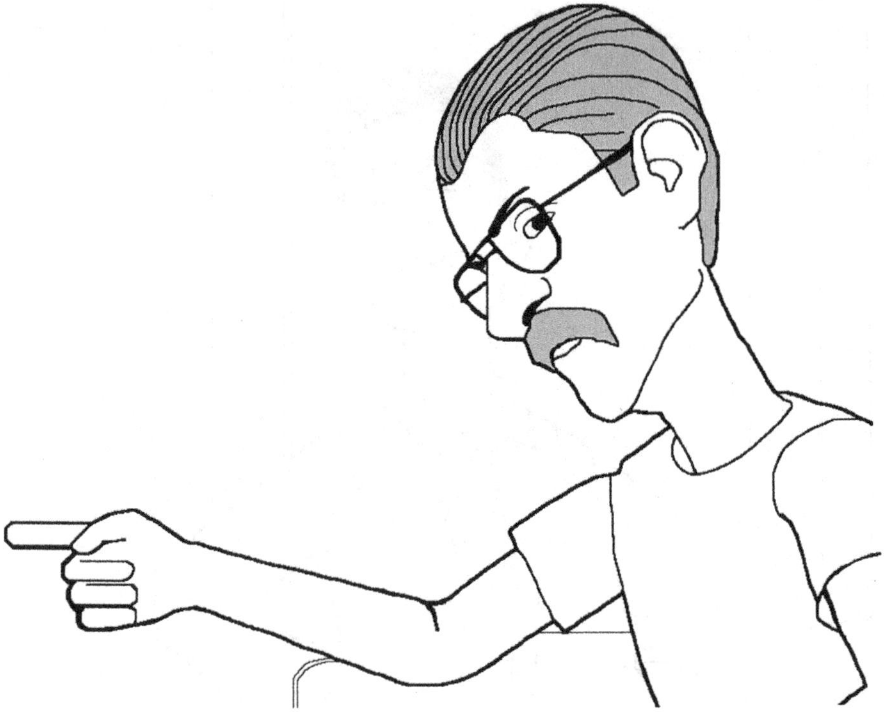

"But you said you were a doctor!" said Dr. Smith.

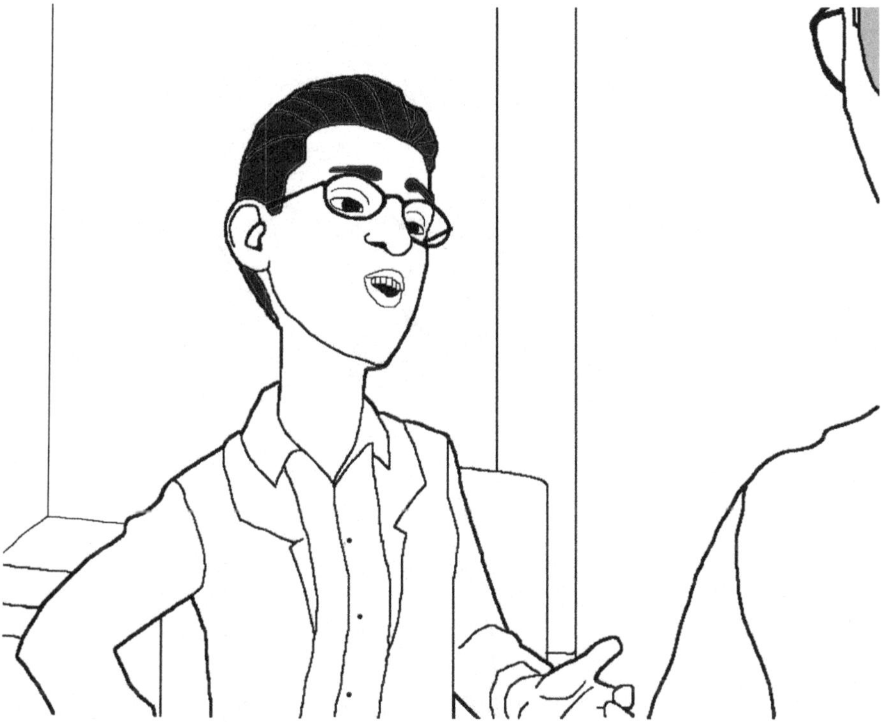

"Yes. I have a Doctorate of Medical Science degree. Physician associates are now getting that degree and are becoming doctors," the physician assistant replied.

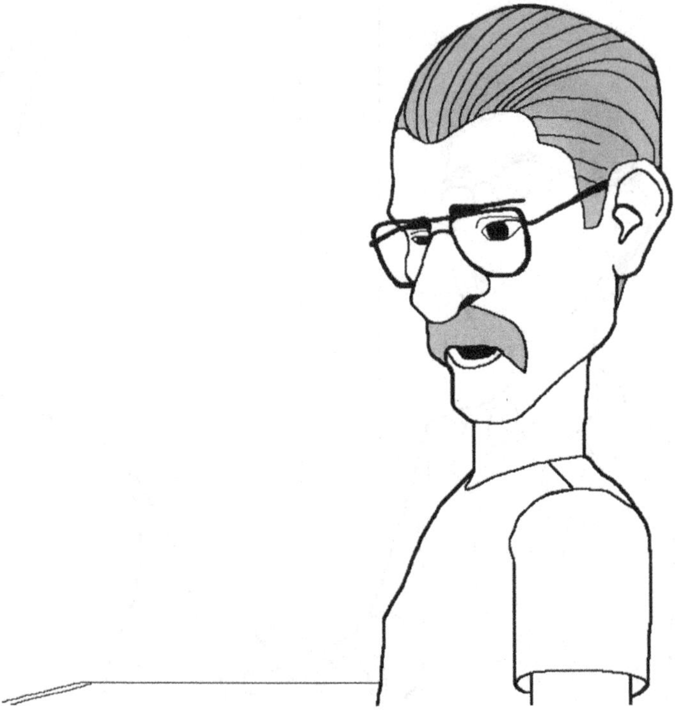

"This is crazy," said Dr. Smith. "When will I get to see a physician? Is the orthopedic surgeon a physician?"

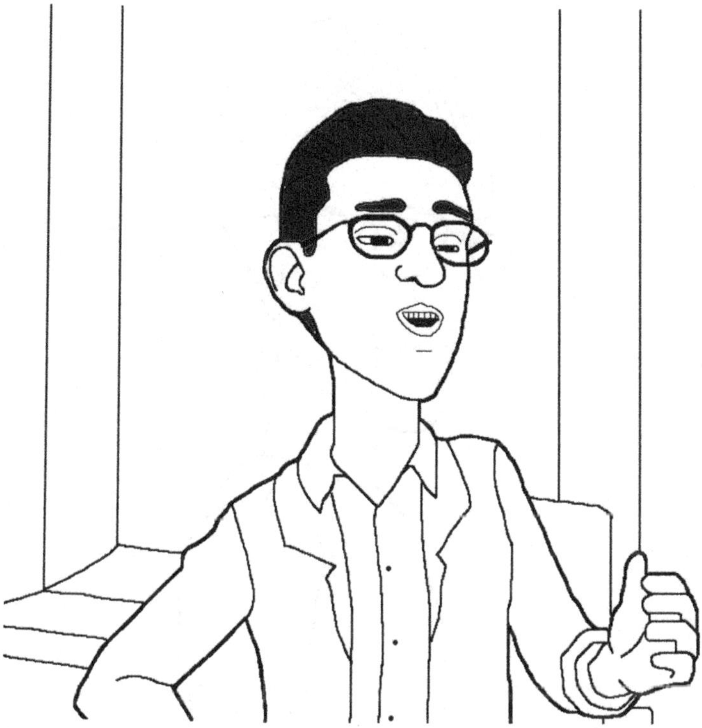

"Yes," he answered. "Although some non-physician practitioners do surgery too."

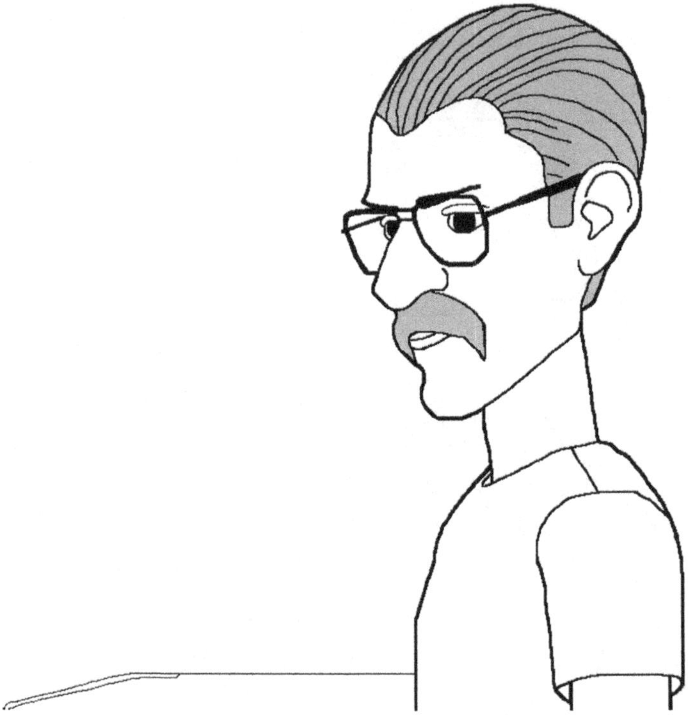

"Great. When do I get to meet the surgeon?" Dr. Smith asked.

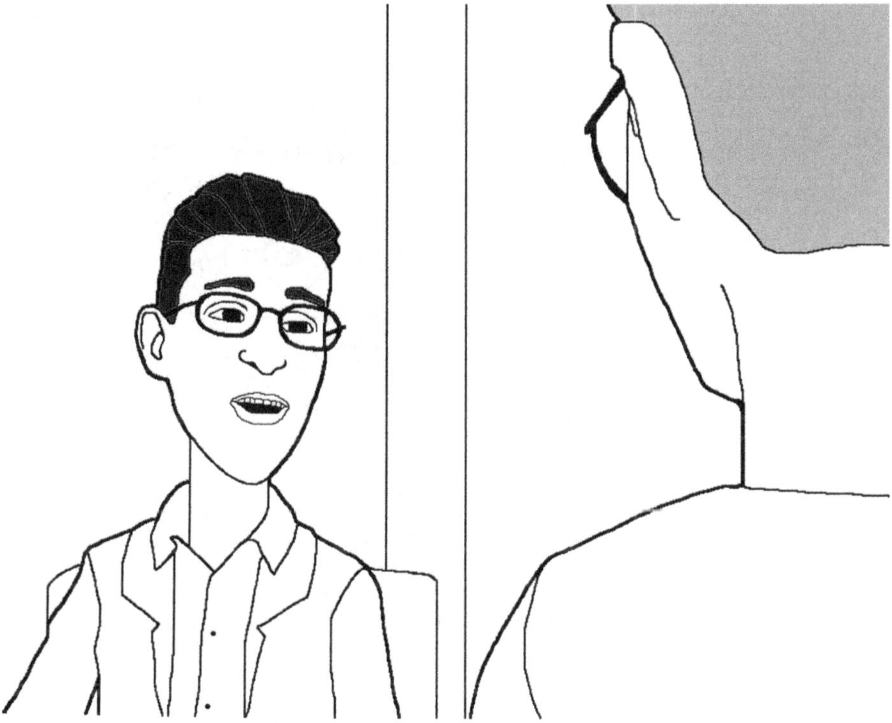

"She will be in the operating room," the physician assistant replied.

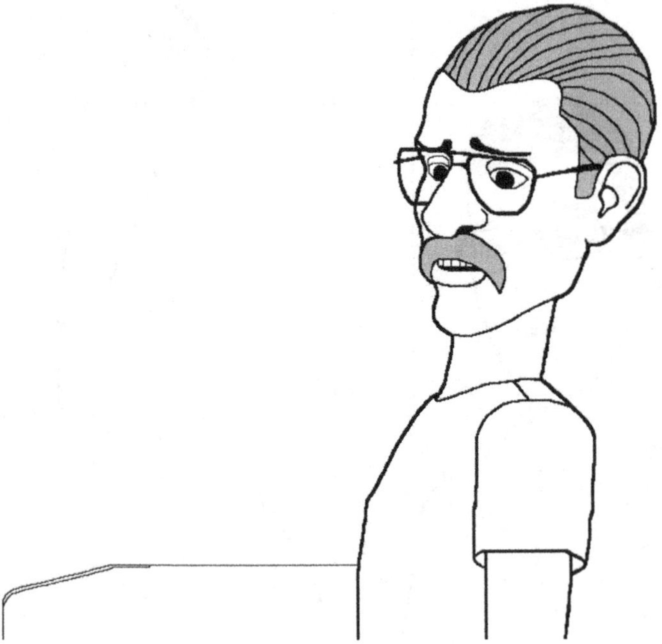

“You mean I don’t get to meet my surgeon until right before the surgery? That’s not right!” Dr. Smith exclaimed.

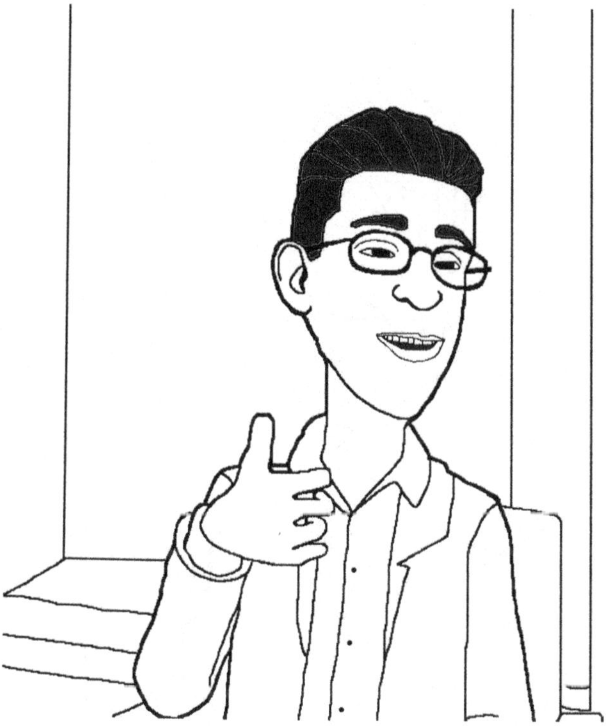

"I will be doing your examination before surgery and will check on you after surgery," said the physician assistant.

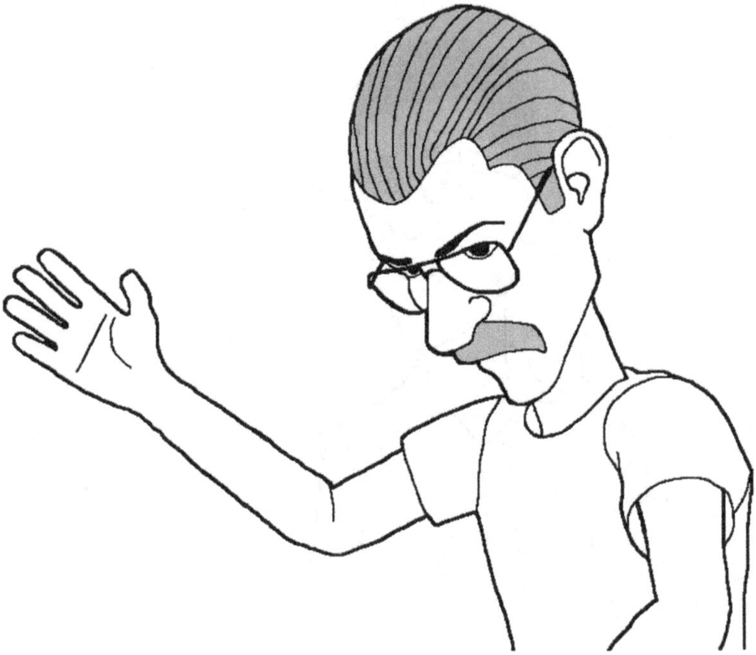

“I am done talking with you. Examine me if you must and give me whatever forms you need signed, but then go away.” Dr. Smith was annoyed.

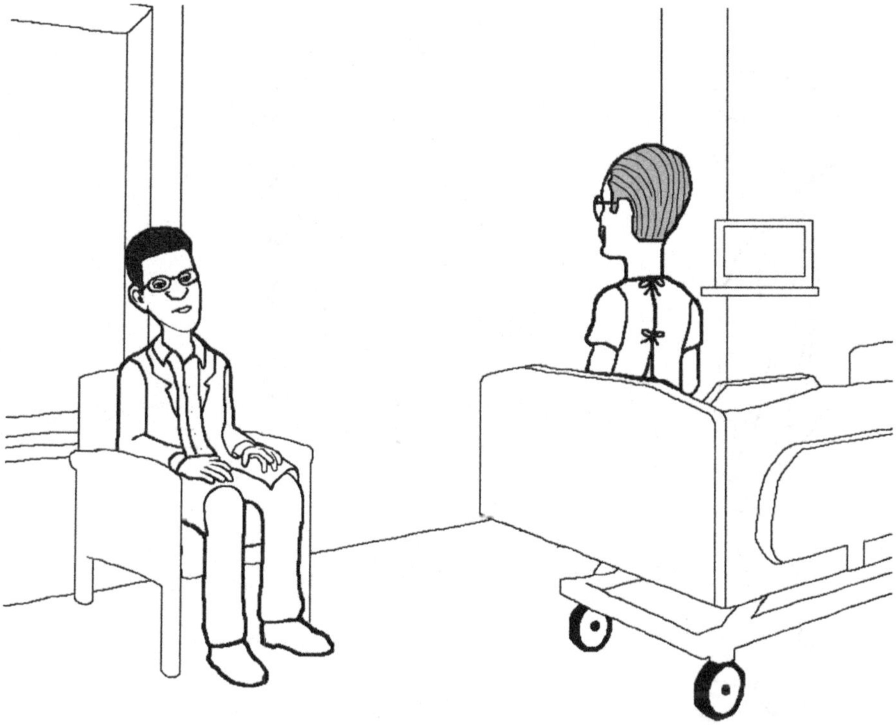

The physician assistant did a quick examination, had Dr. Smith sign some papers, and left the room.

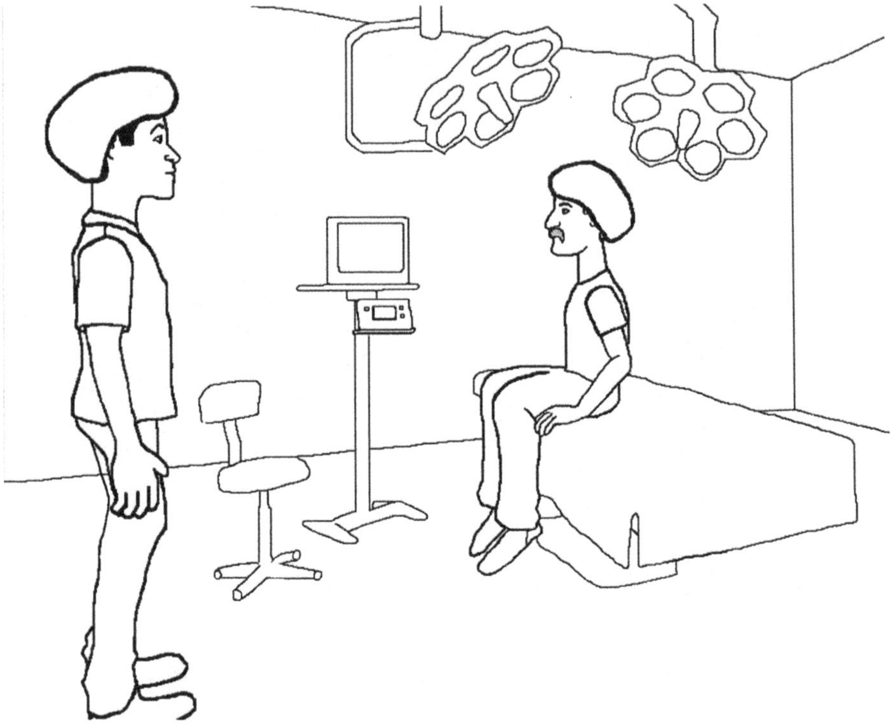

Dr. Smith was taken to the operating room a few hours later. A man wearing scrubs greeted him.

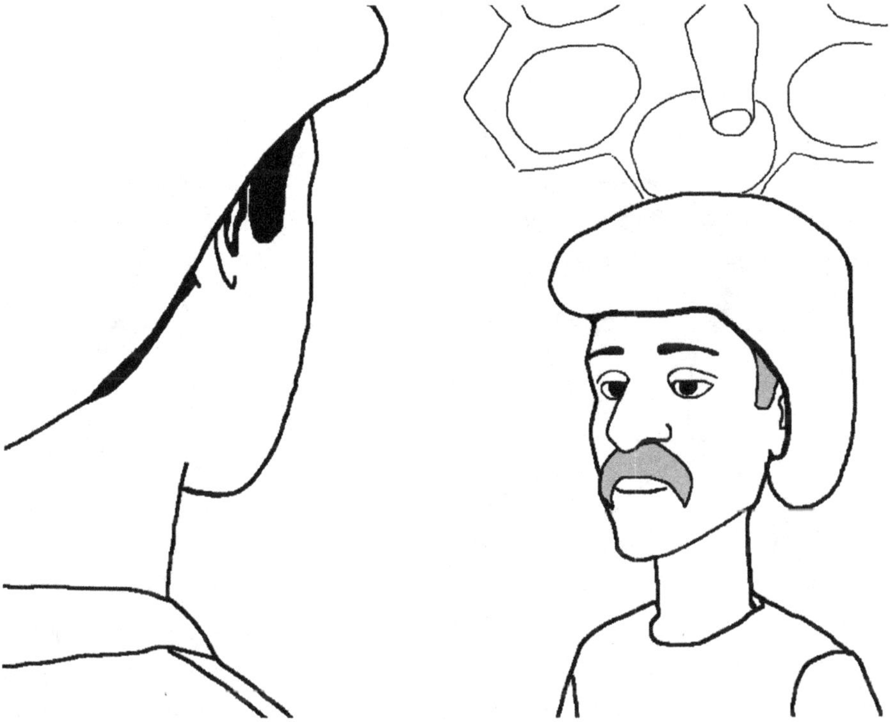

“Are you a physician?” asked Dr. Smith.

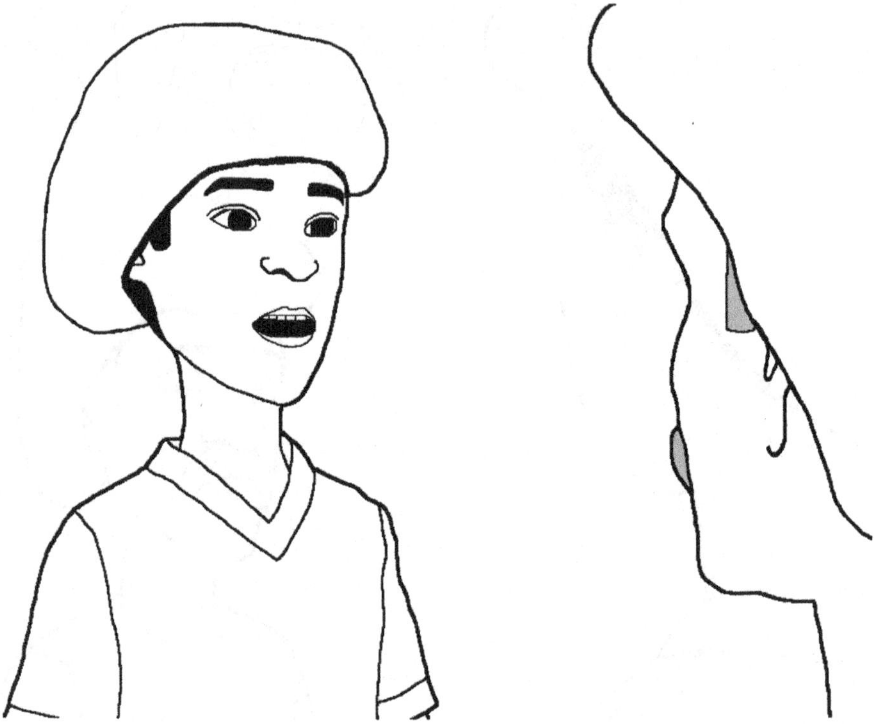

"No," he replied. "I am a CRNA or nurse anesthetist. I will be doing the anesthesia for your hip surgery."

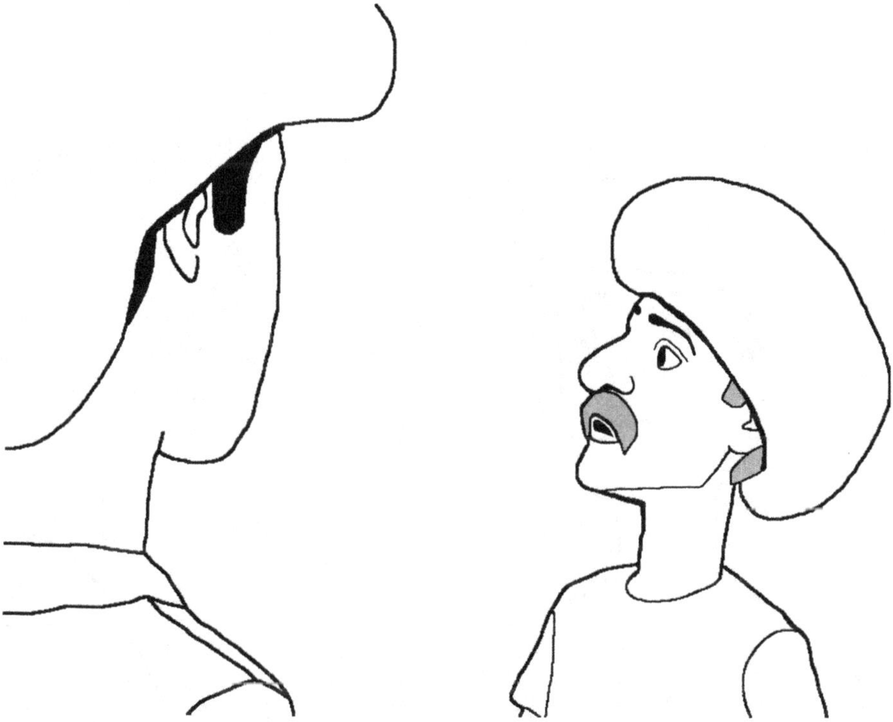

"Where is the anesthesiologist?" asked Dr. Smith, looking around.

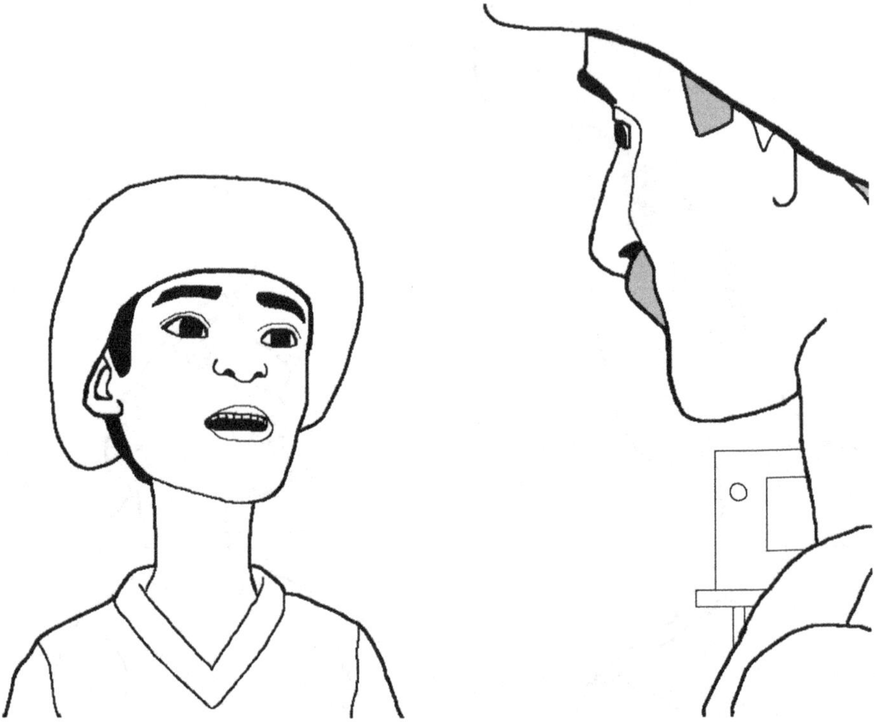

“There is one anesthesiologist supervising all the CRNAs,” the nurse anesthetist replied. “He doesn’t come into the operating rooms unless there is a problem.”

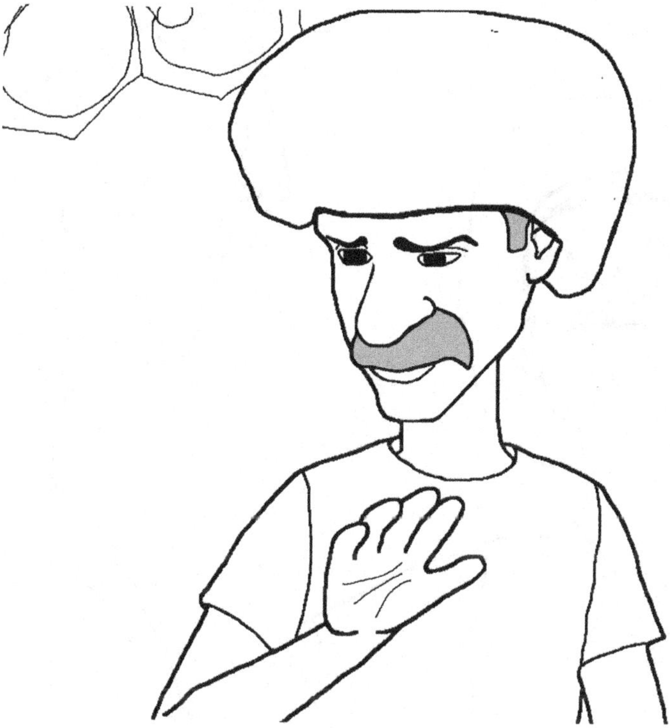

Dr. Smith could not believe what he was hearing.

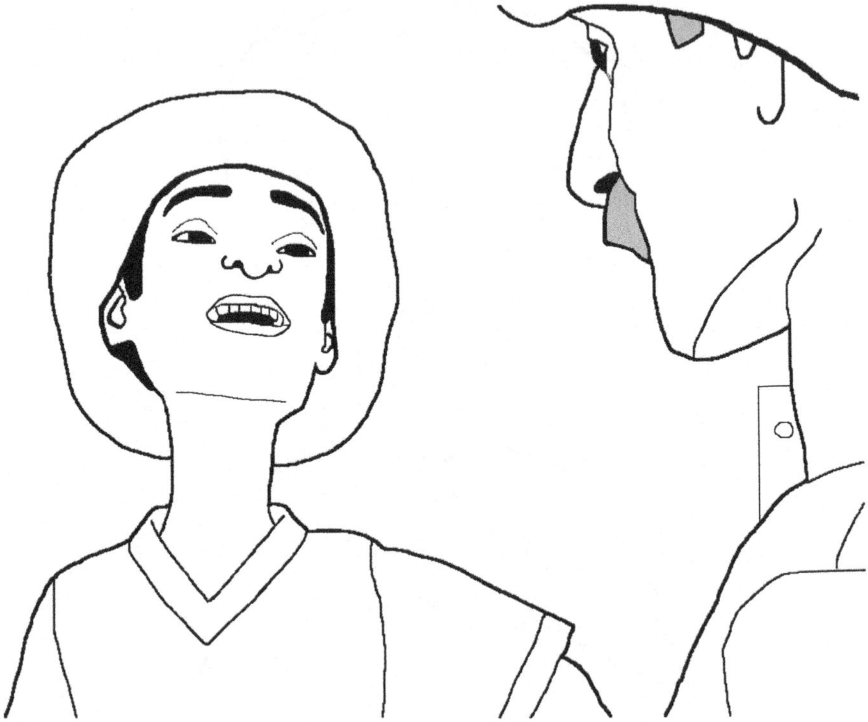

“Don’t worry,” the nurse anesthetist said. “I am fully capable of doing the anesthesia for your hip surgery.”

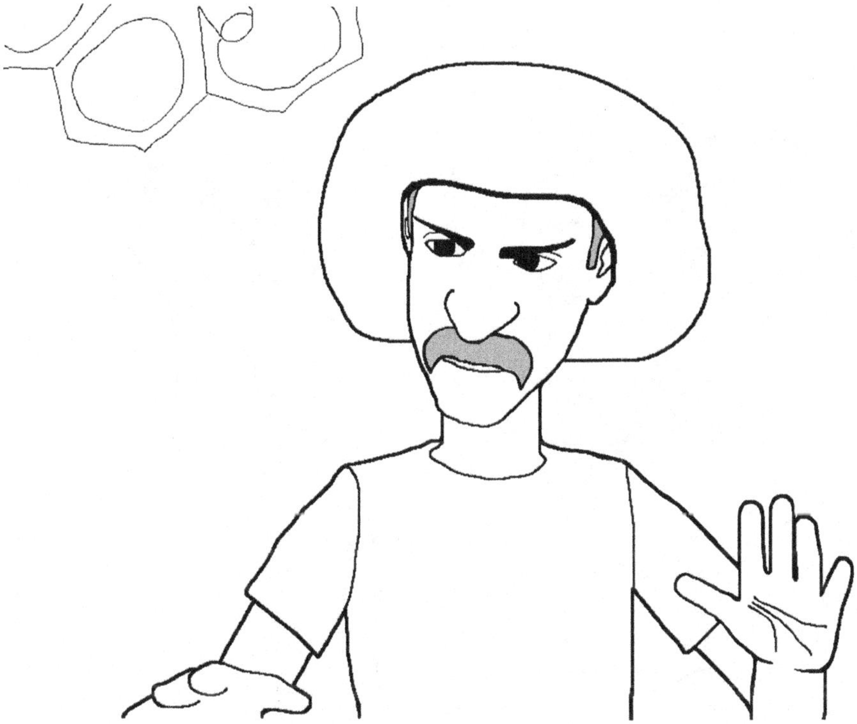

"I feel like I am in a bad dream," said Dr. Smith, shaking his head.

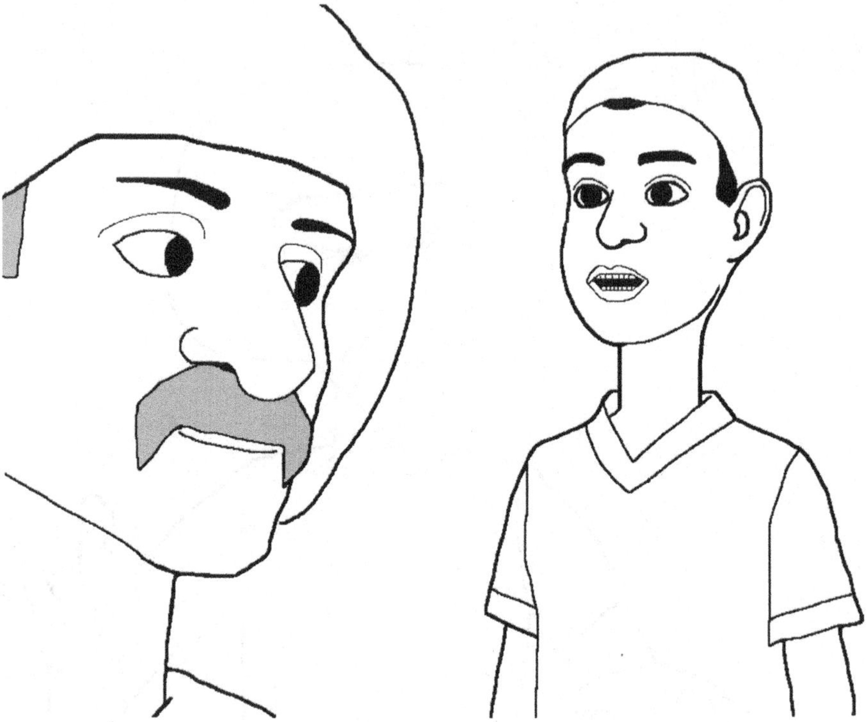

A woman in scrubs appeared behind Dr. Smith. “Is this the patient with the left hip fracture?” she asked.

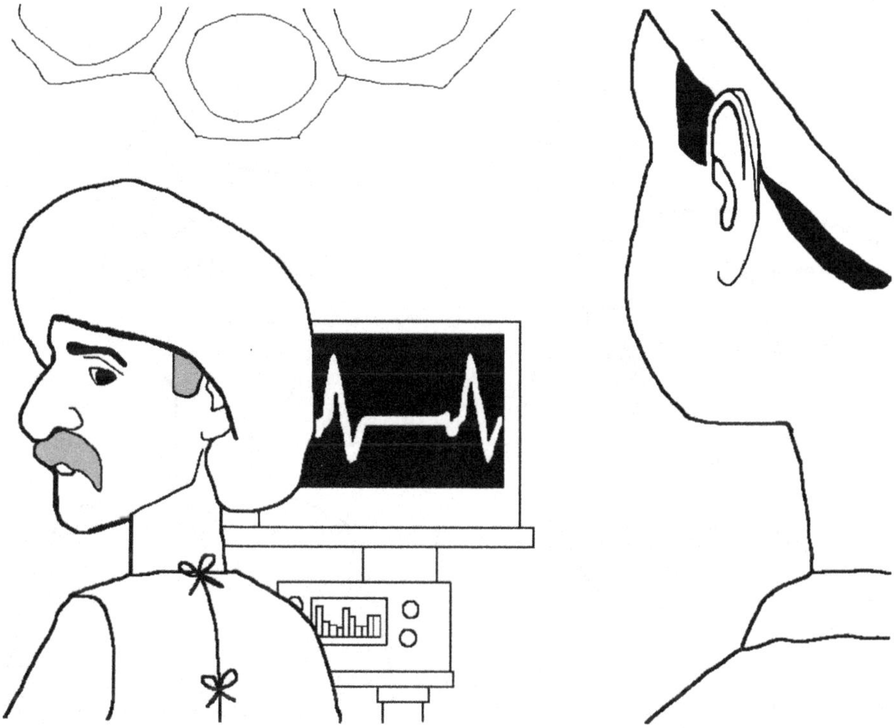

"Are you the orthopedic surgeon?" Dr. Smith asked her.

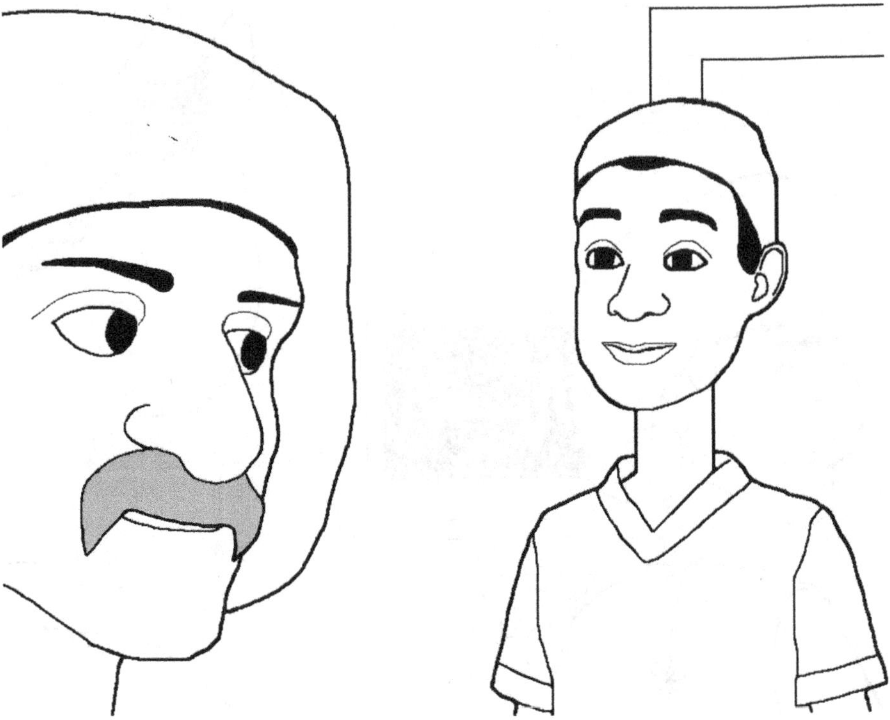

“Yes, she replied. “I am Dr. Leonard.”

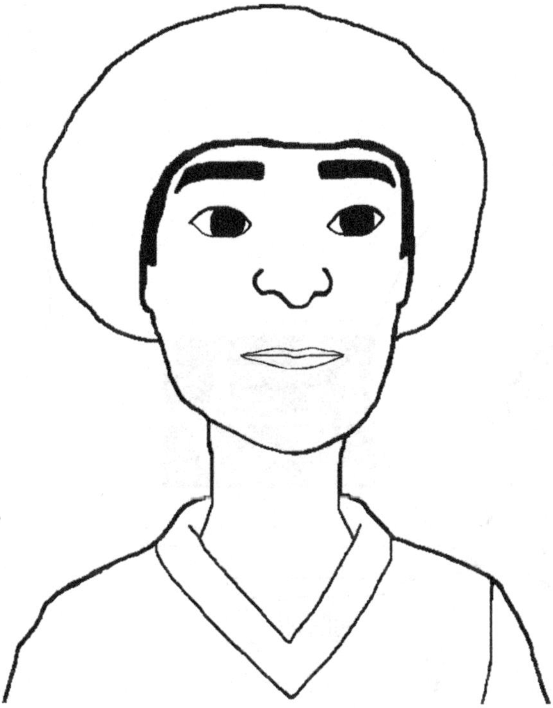

“Doctor,” interrupted the nurse anesthetist, “you have three other surgical cases today. I will get this patient anesthetized right away. The physician assistant has already obtained consent for surgery.”

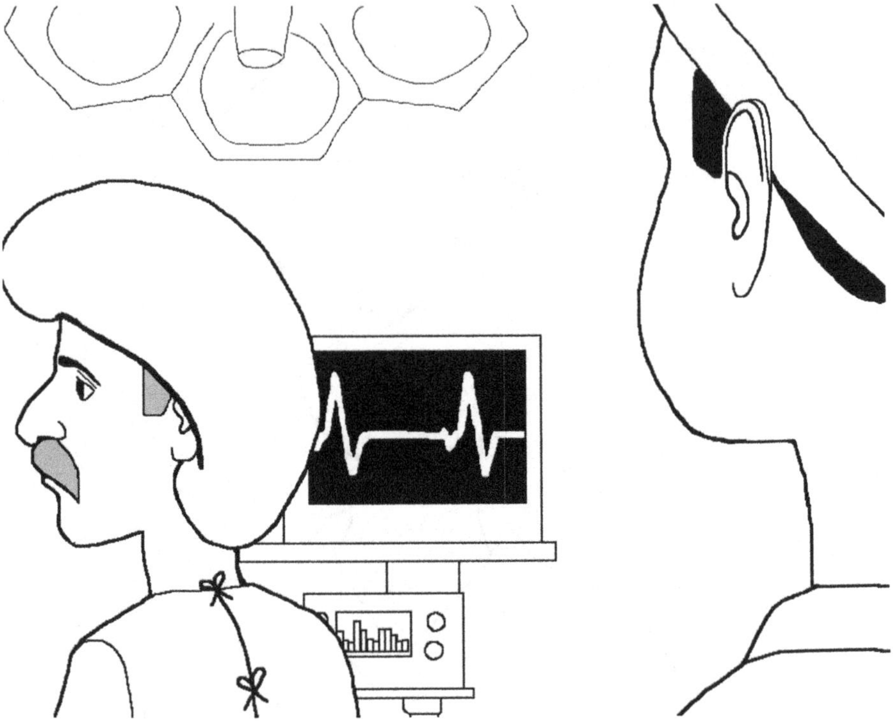

“Okay,” said Dr Leonard and left the operating room.

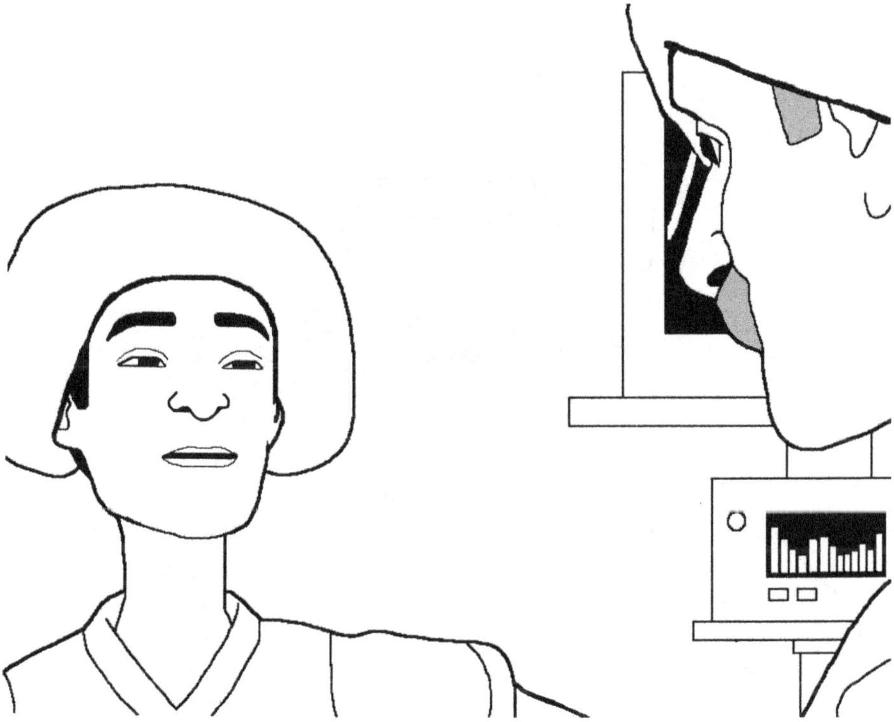

“I need to put you under anesthesia for surgery now,” said the nurse anesthetist.

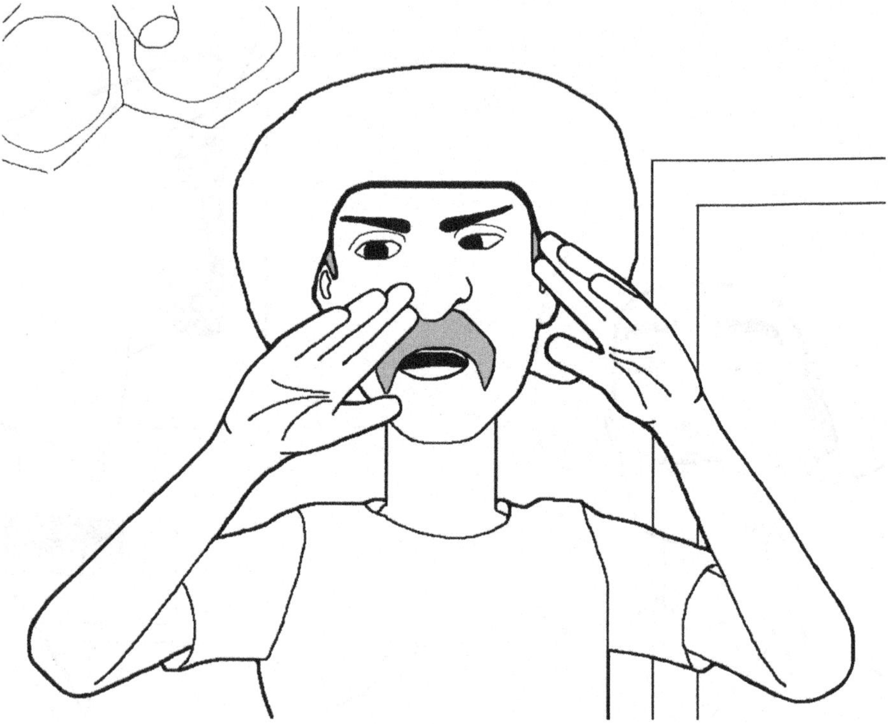

“But I haven’t spoken with the surgeon yet,” said Dr. Smith. “This isn’t right!”

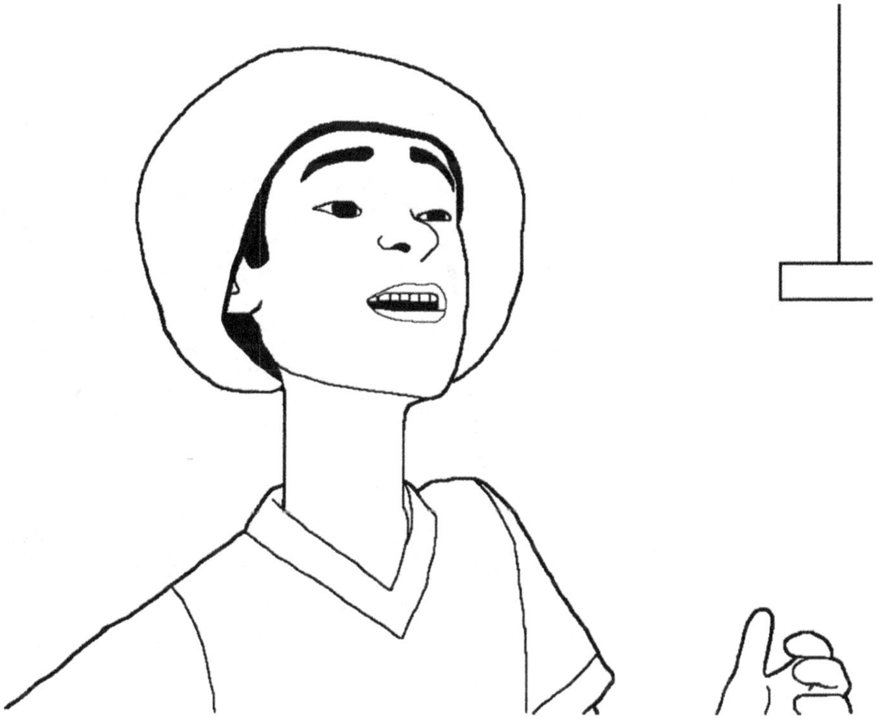

"Goodnight. Take slow deep breaths and you will wake up when the surgery is done," said the nurse anesthetist.

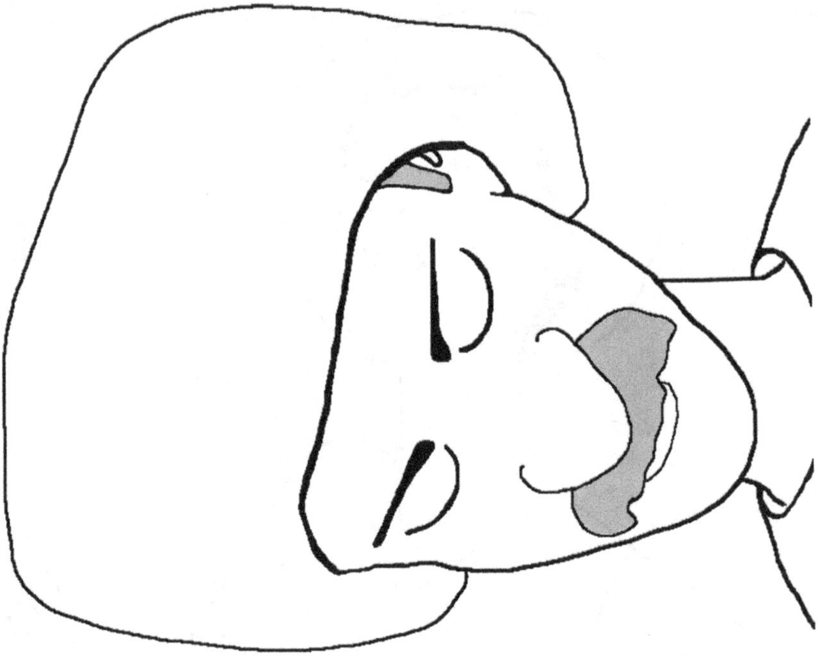

"But... wait..." said Dr. Smith, as he fell asleep.

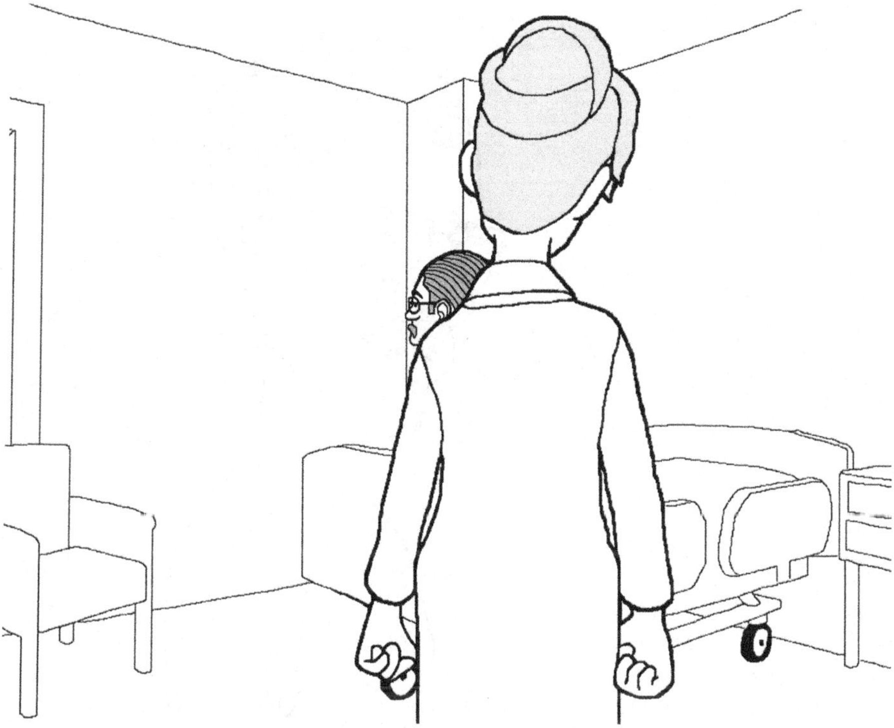

Dr. Smith woke up in his hospital room the next morning. A woman wearing a white coat entered the room and introduced herself as Dr. O'Malley.

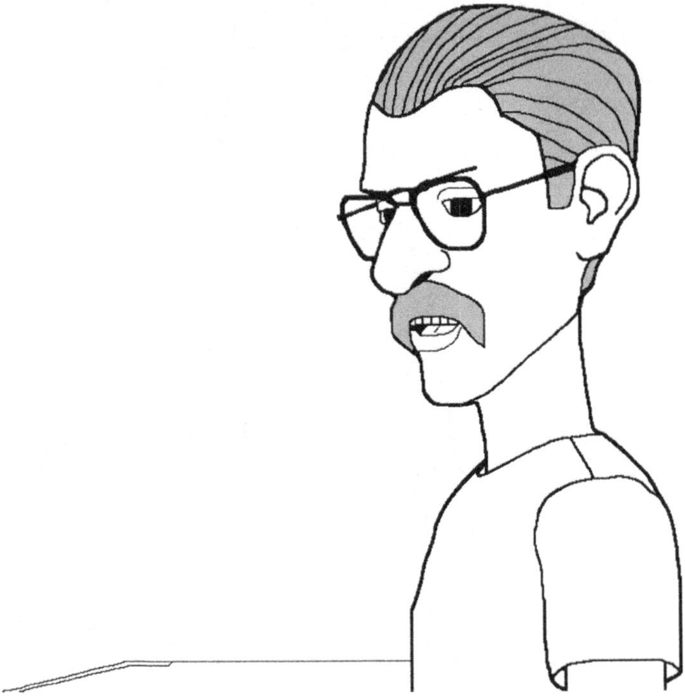

"Are you a physician?" asked Dr. Smith.

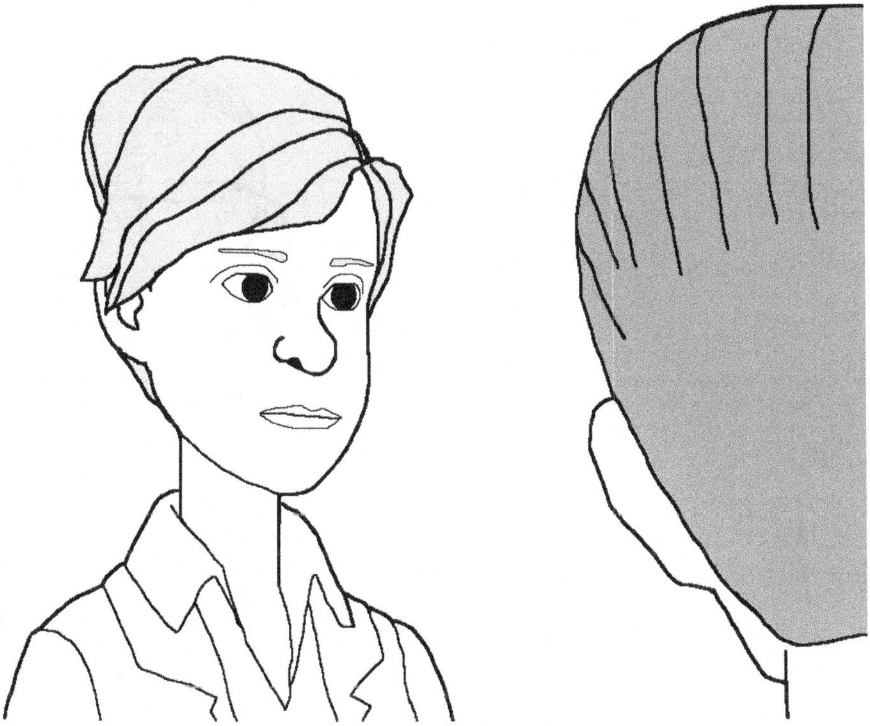

"No," she answered. "I am a physical therapist. I am here to get you moving around after surgery."

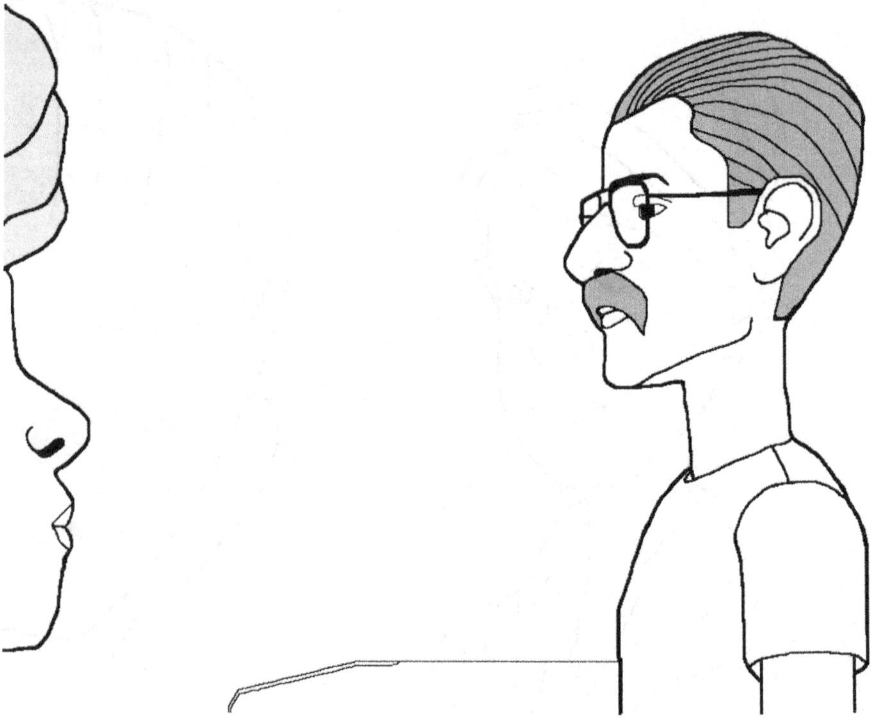

“I am confused,” Dr. Smith said. “You said you were a doctor?”

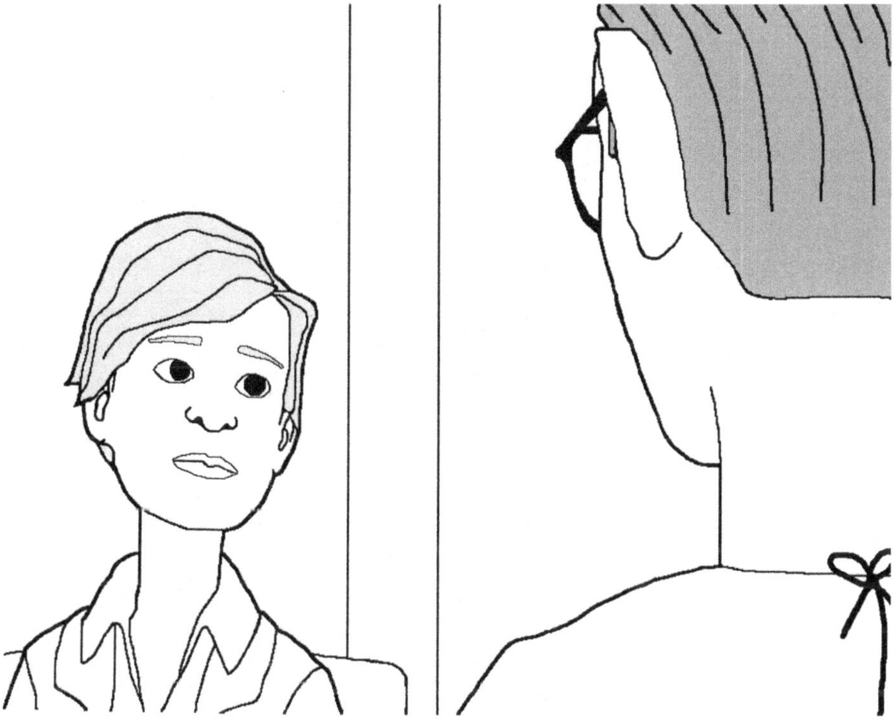

“I have a doctorate degree in physical therapy,” she answered. “Now let’s get you out of that bed and into a chair.”

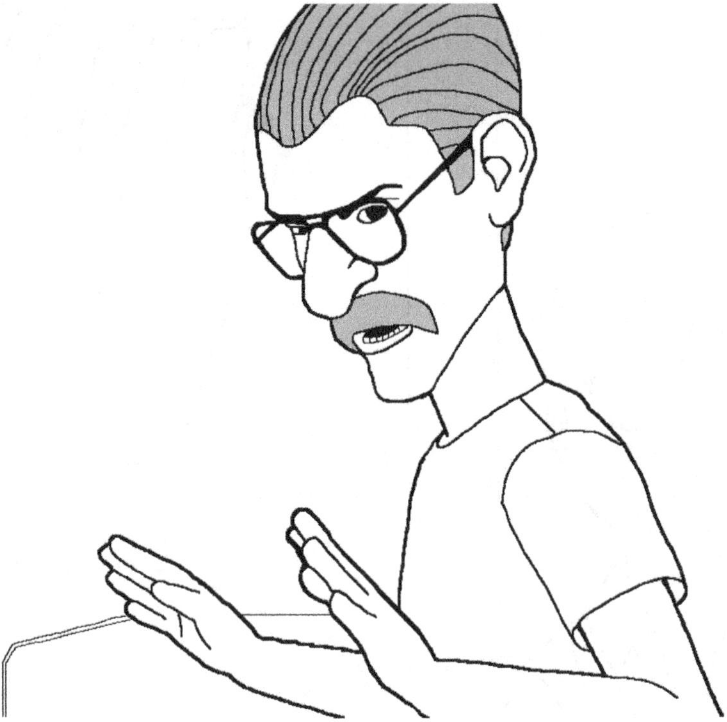

“Everyone here is a doctor but almost no one is a physician!” grunted Dr. Smith.

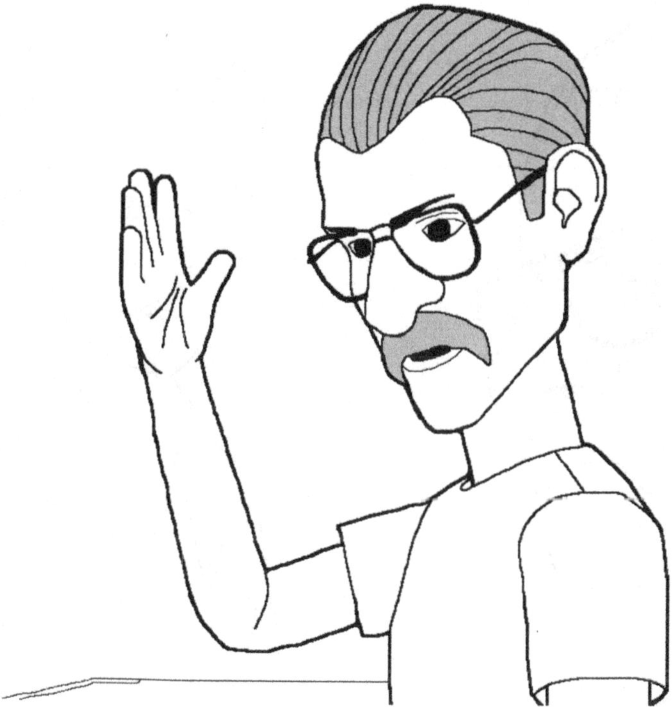

"Get out of my room and send in the orthopedic surgeon. I barely said hello to her before my surgery and I want to know how long I have to stay in this crazy hospital before I can go home." Dr. Smith was getting angry.

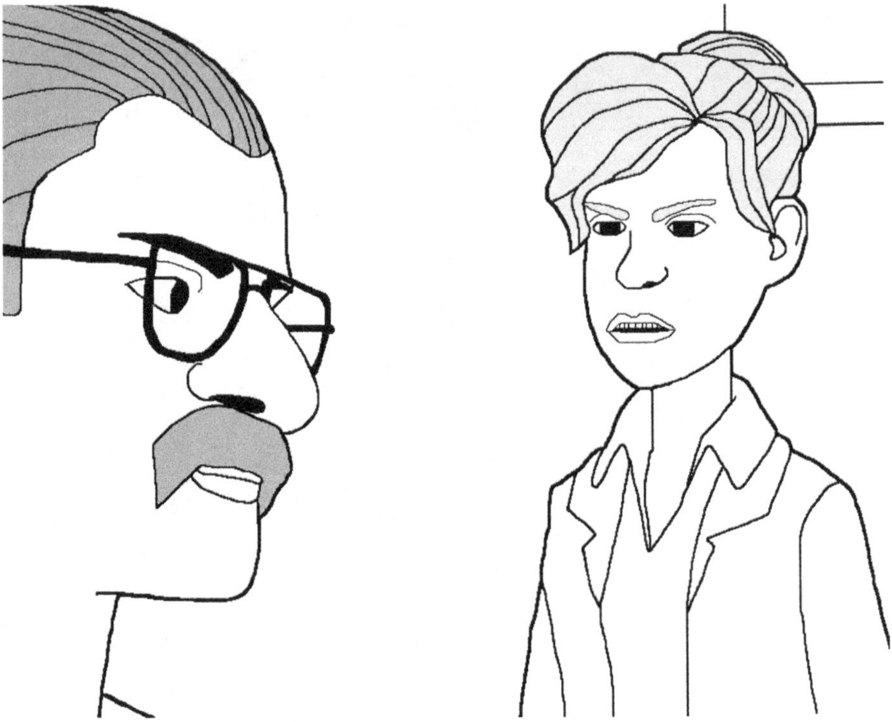

"I don't know why you are getting so upset," said the physical therapist.

Dr. Smith just looked away. He had nothing more to say.

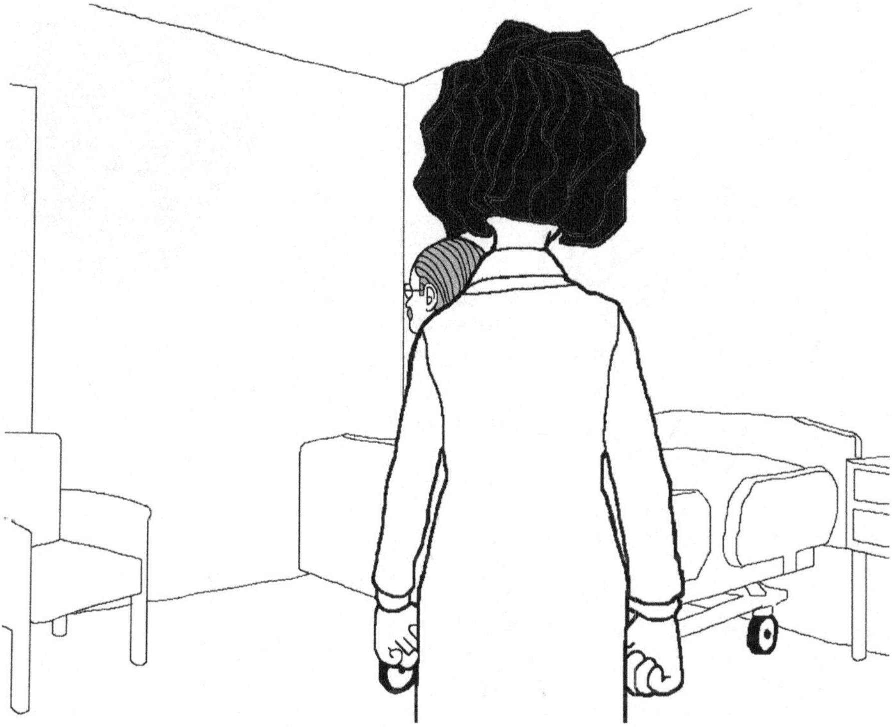

A woman wearing a white coat entered the room a little while later.

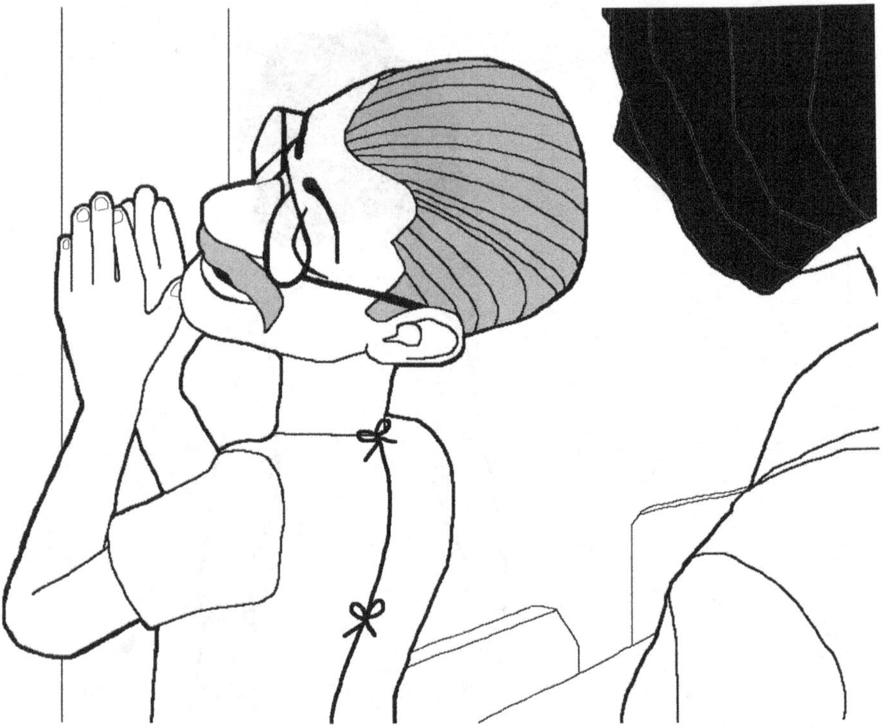

"Are you one of the orthopedic surgeons?" asked Dr. Smith.

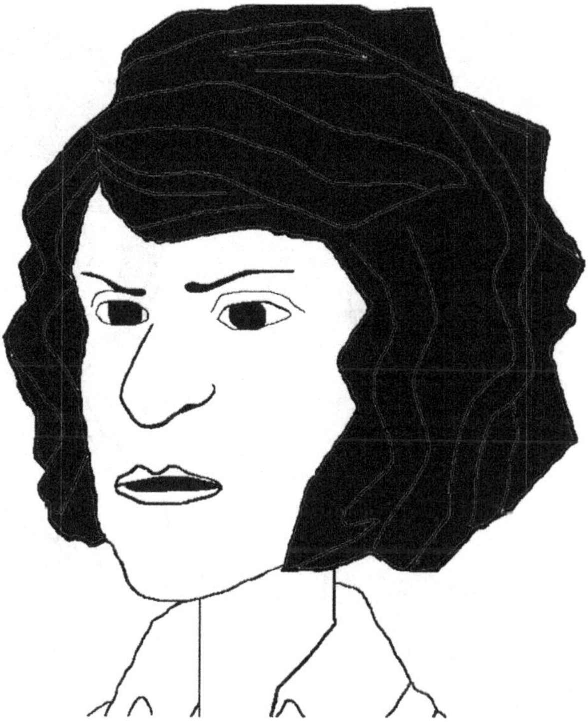

"No," she said, "I am Dr. Amari. I would like to speak with you."

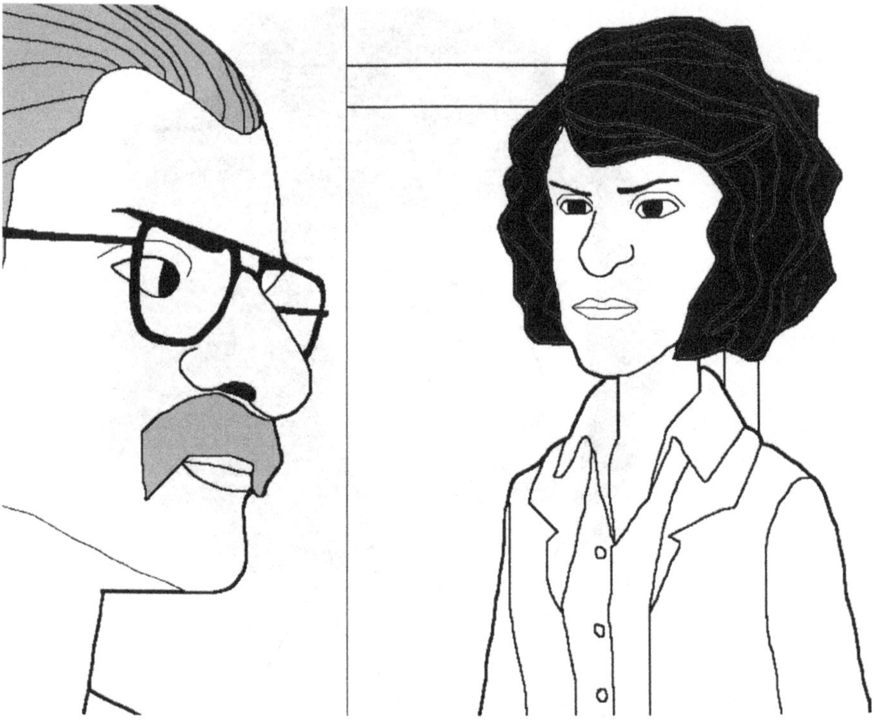

"Are you a physician?" asked Dr. Smith.

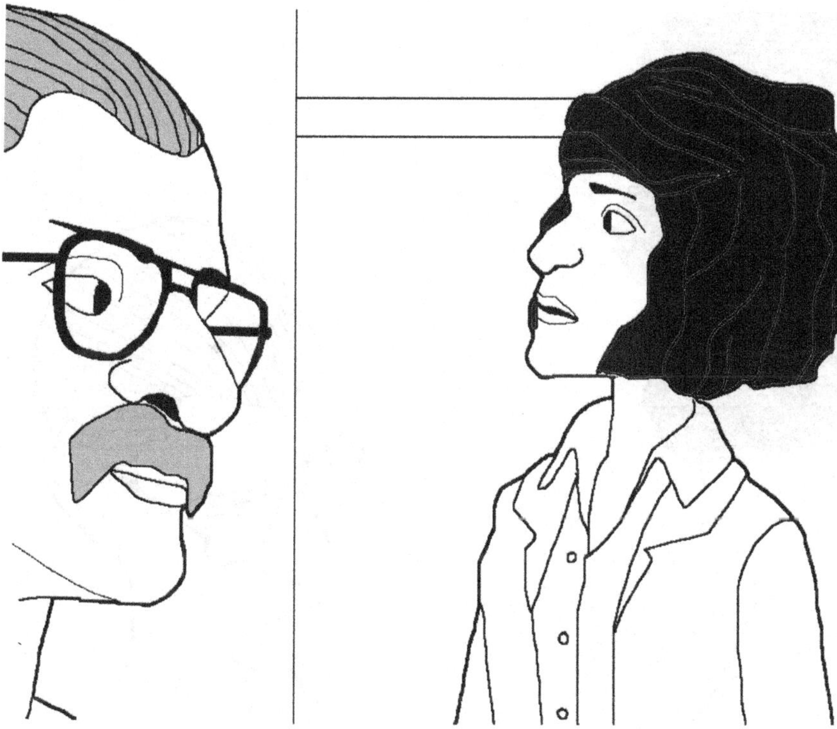

"No, she answered and looked around the room. "I am a psychologist. I would like to talk with you to find out why you are not cooperating with the hospital staff."

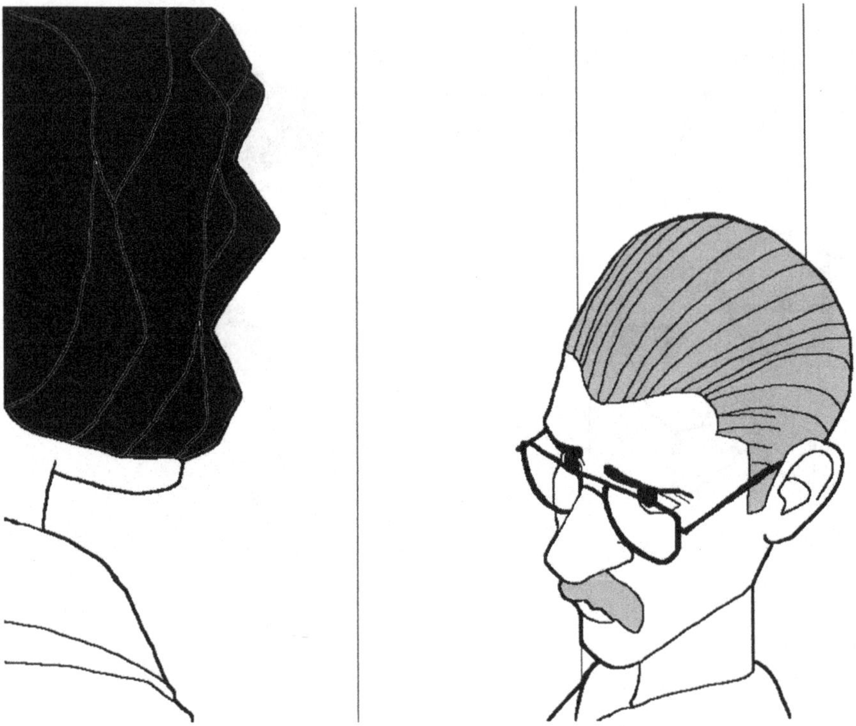

"You said you were a doctor," said Dr. Smith, looking over his glasses at her.

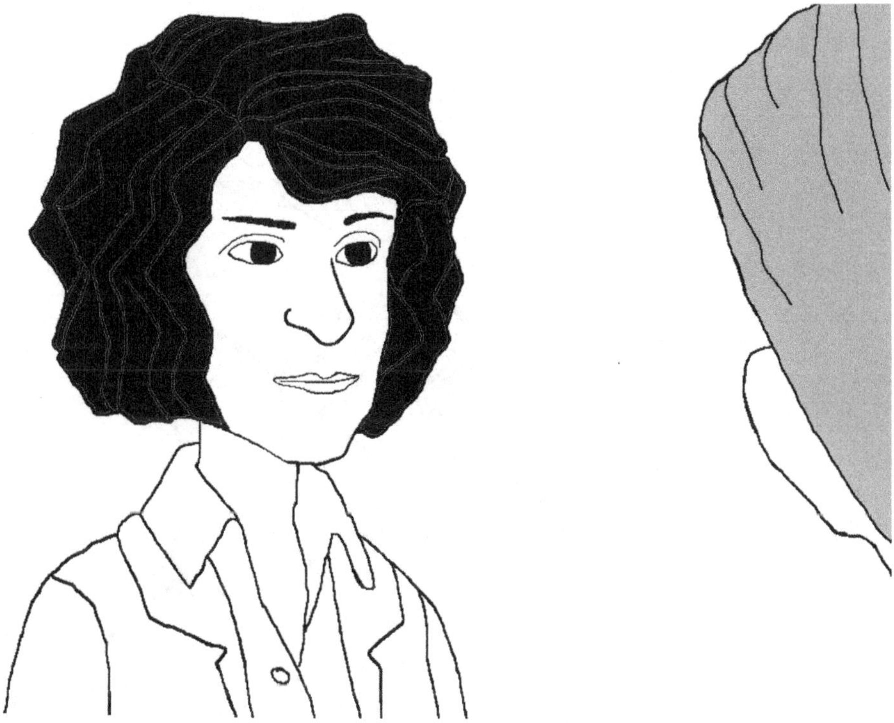

“Yes,” the psychologist said. “I have a PsyD degree. May I sit down and talk with you?”

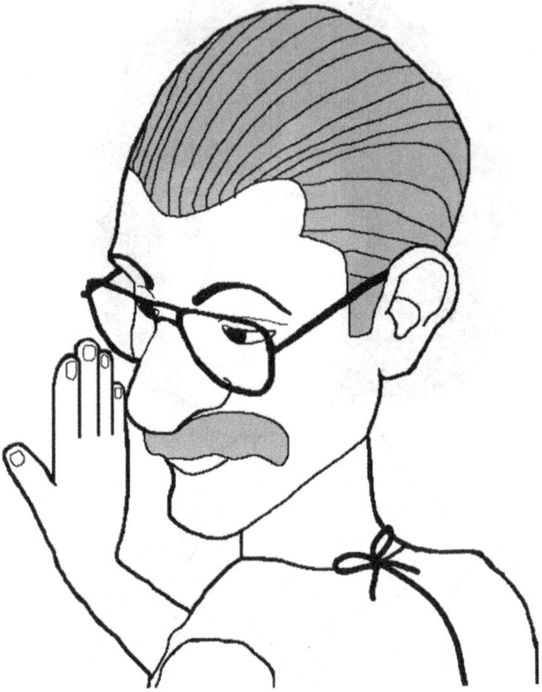

"I have nothing to say to you or anyone else," said Dr. Smith. "Get me the forms to sign so that I can leave the hospital."

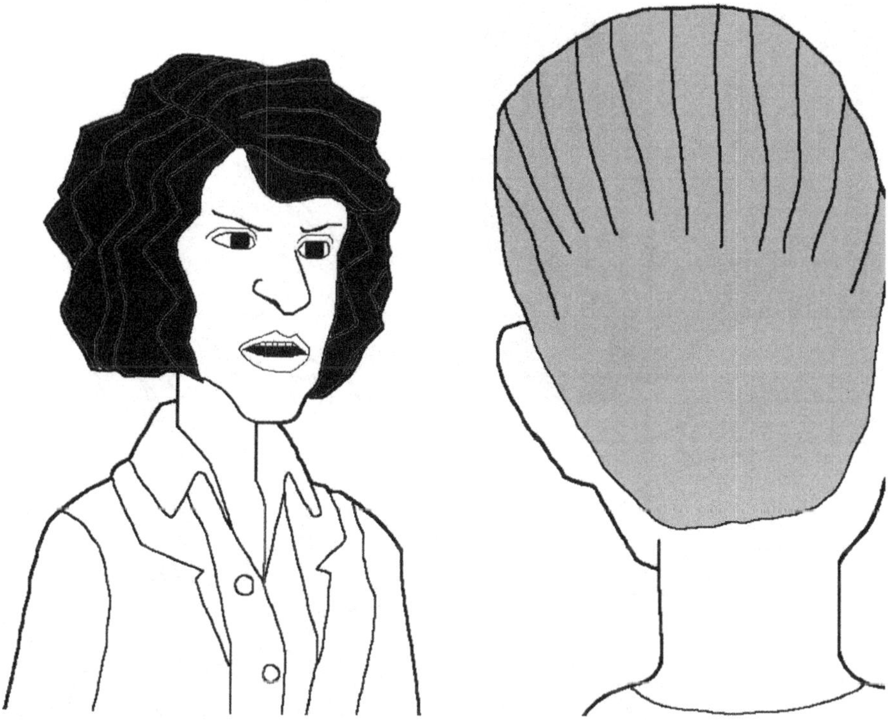

"Do you really think that is a good idea?" asked the psychologist.

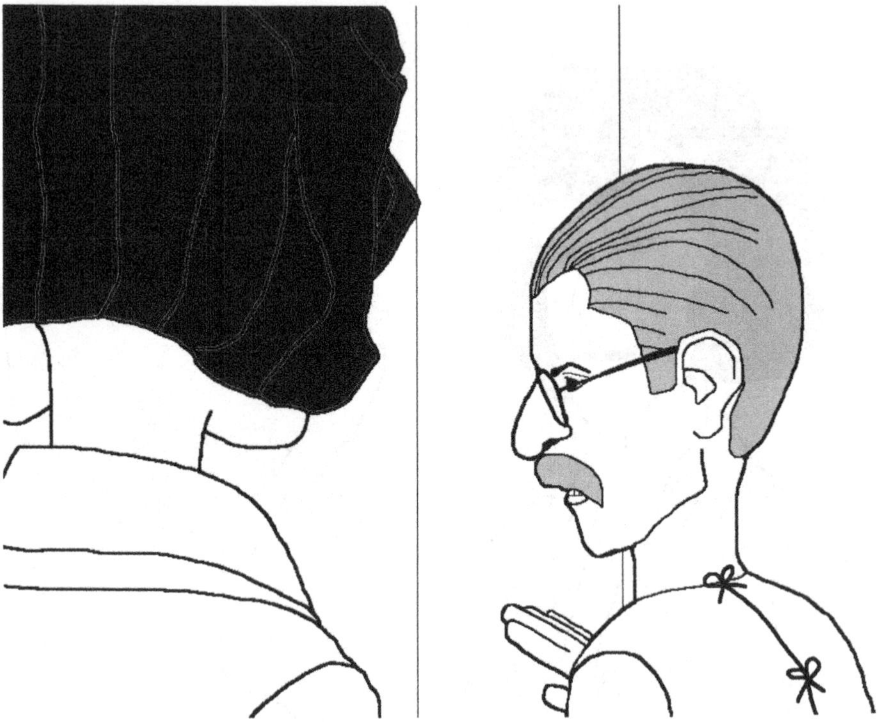

"No," said Dr. Smith, "but I will follow up with my family physician. She is a real doctor. Apparently, real doctors are like unicorns in this hospital."

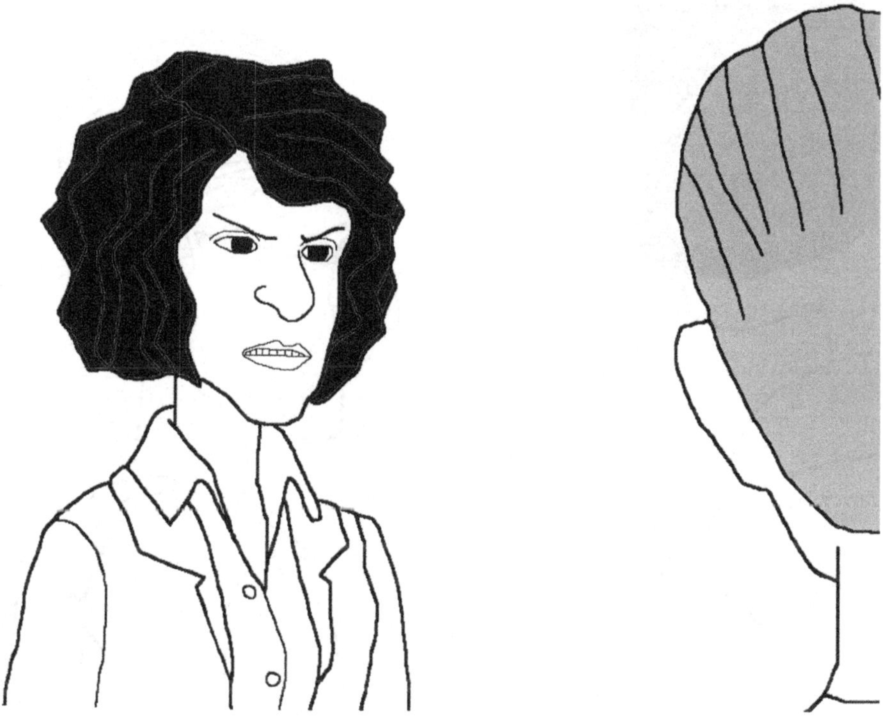

"I think you are making a big mistake," said the psychologist.

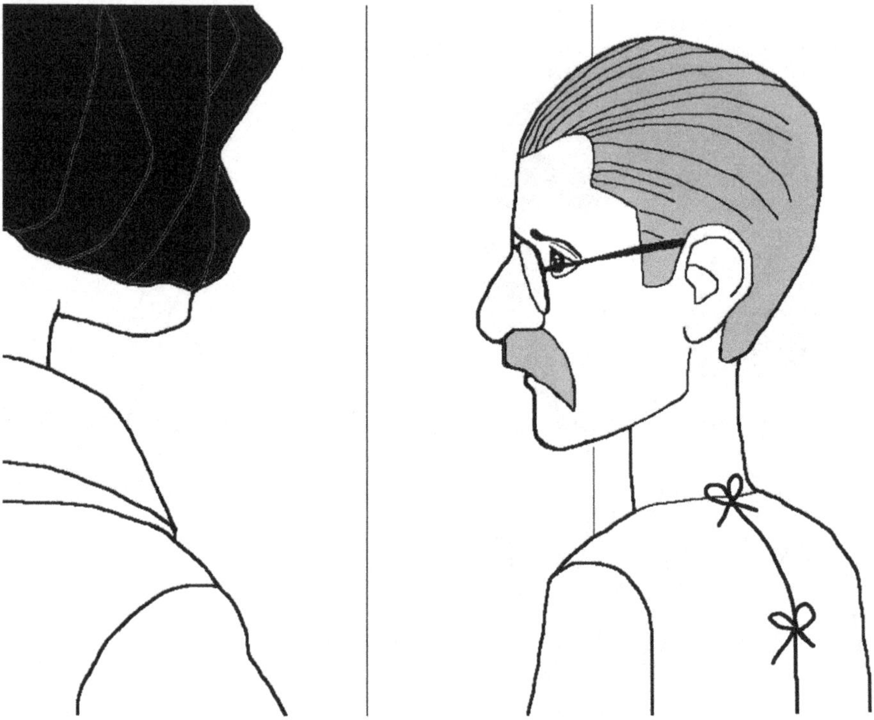

"Go away!" said Dr. Smith.

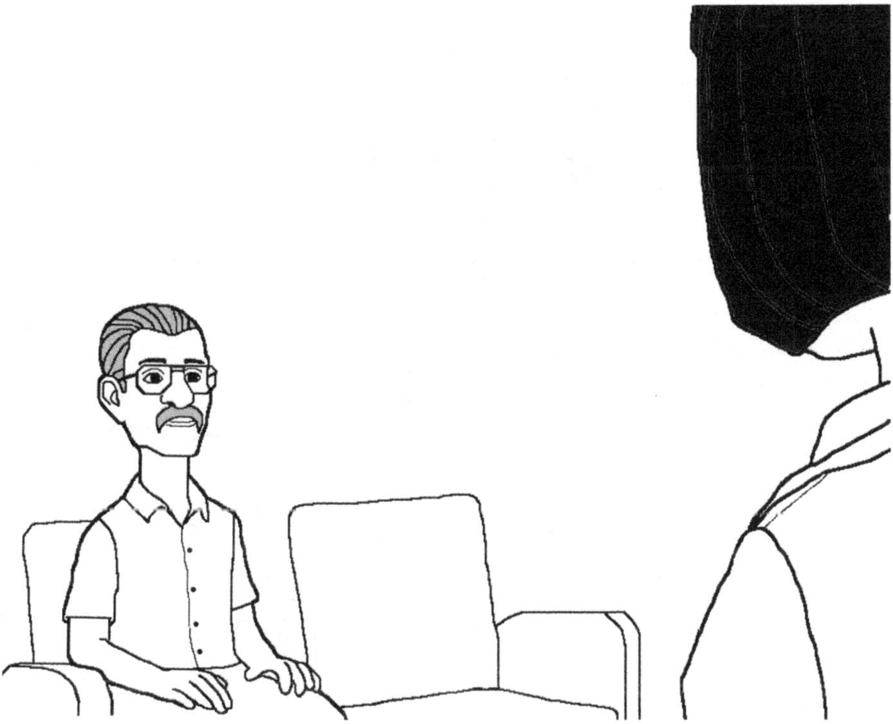

Dr. Smith signed himself out of the hospital. He went to see his family physician that same day.

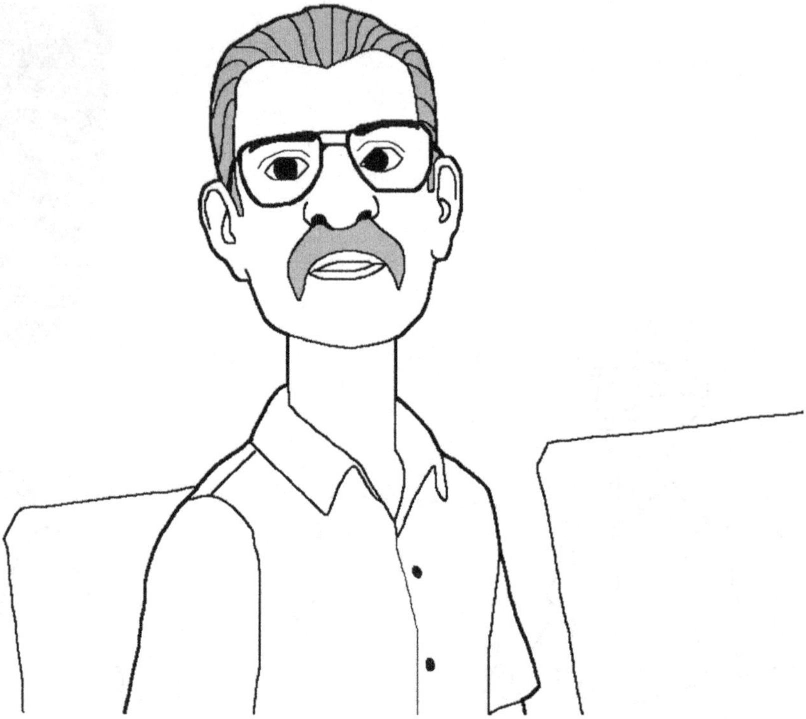

"Oh, Dr. Green," said Dr. Smith. "You have no idea what the last couple of days have been like."

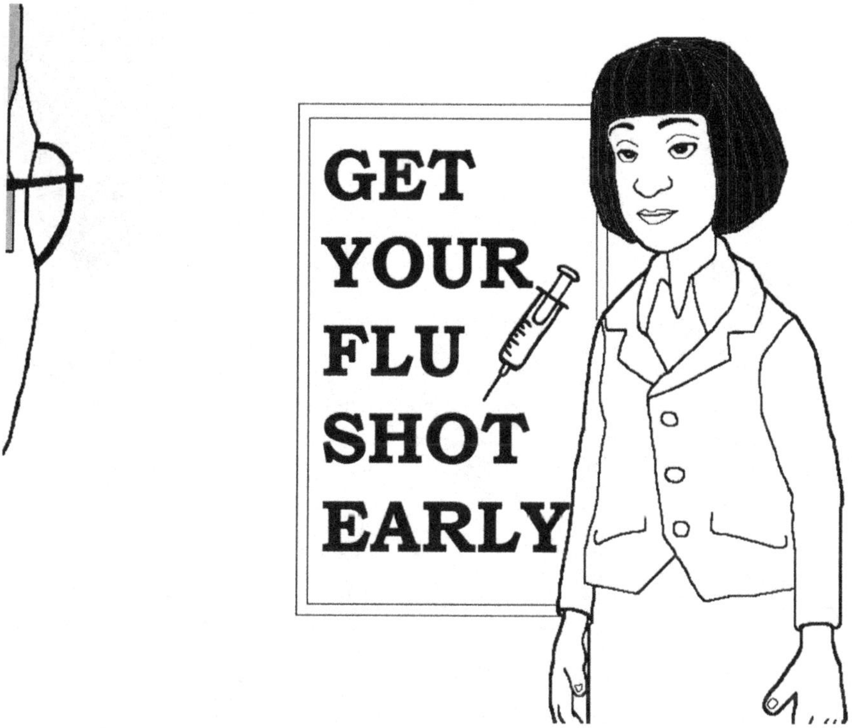

"I heard you broke your hip," said Dr. Green. "Shouldn't you still be in the hospital?"

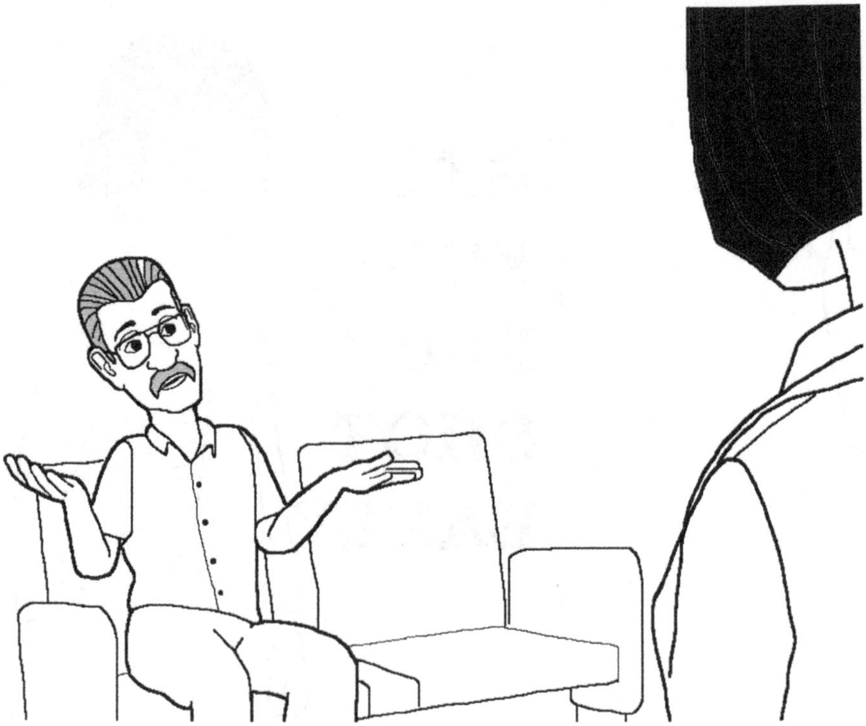

"What for?" asked Dr. Smith. "I was seen by a non-physician doctor in the emergency room. I had my preoperative evaluation done by a non-physician doctor."

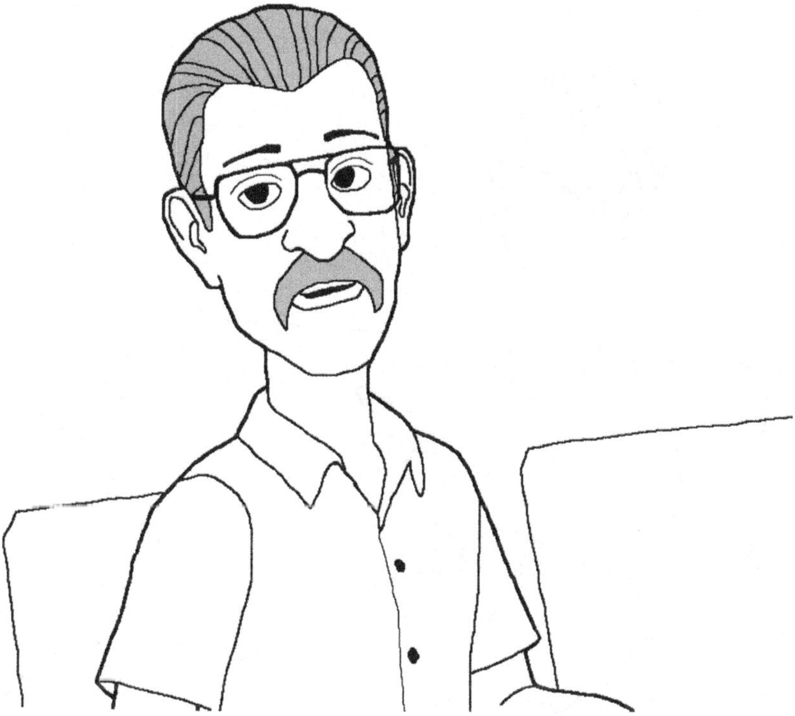

"I had my anesthesia done by a non-physician. My surgery was supposedly done by an orthopedic surgeon and I didn't see her the next day."

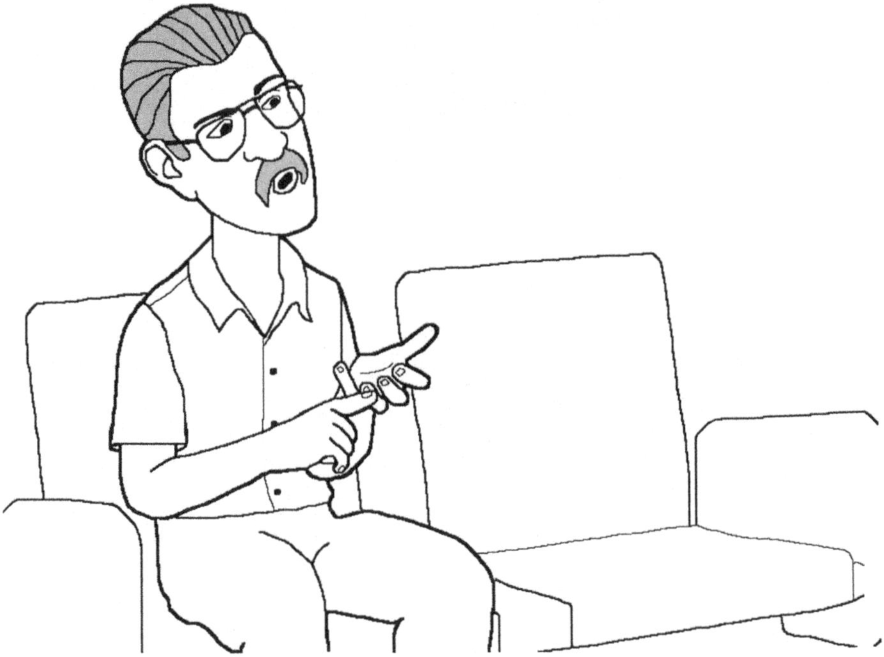

"I saw a non-physician doctor of pharmacy, a non-physician doctor of physical therapy, and a non-physician doctor of psychology. Almost everyone in that hospital is a doctor, but very few are physicians. If this is what medicine has come to, we are doomed!"

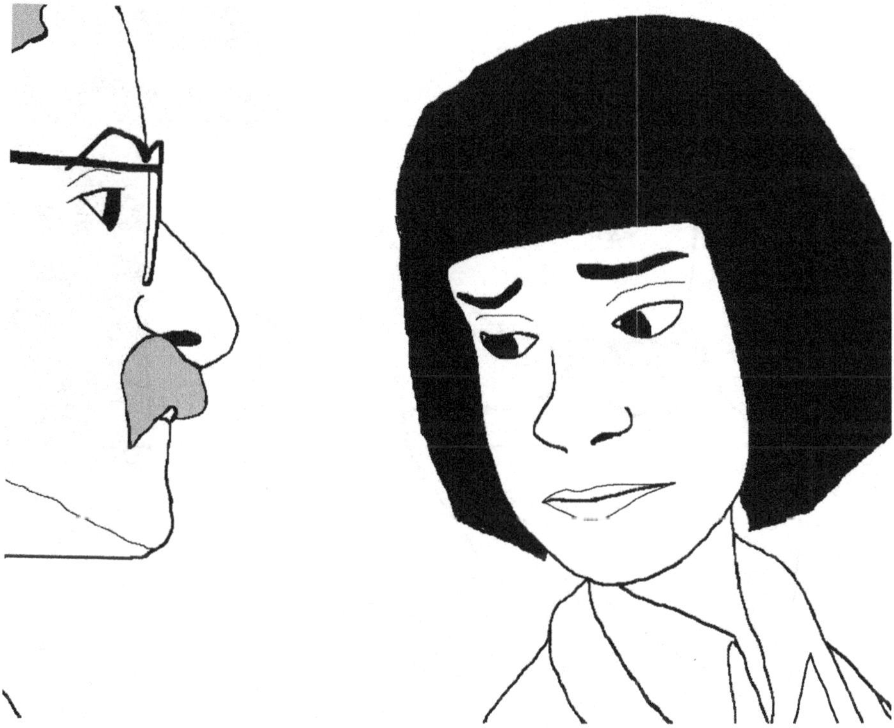

"I am so sorry to hear that you had such a horrible experience," said Dr. Green.

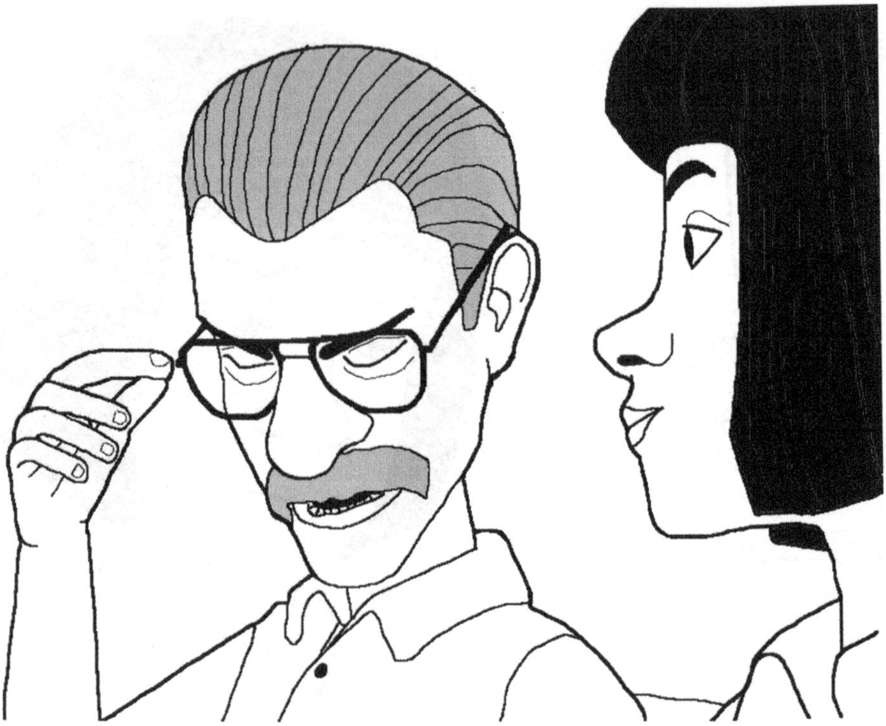

"I'm just happy that I was doing well enough to get out of there," said Dr. Smith.

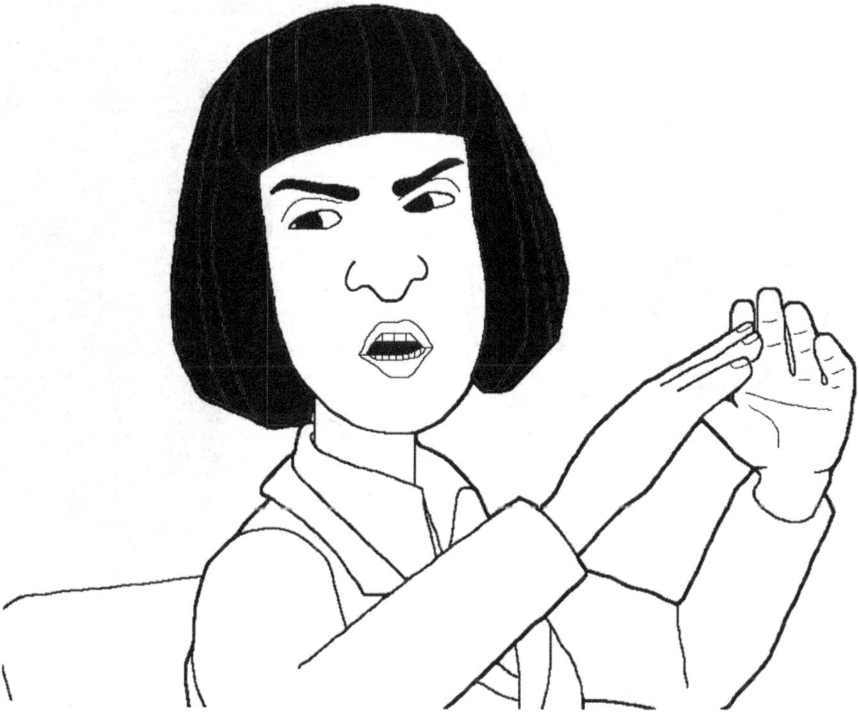

"I will be telling all my patients to stay away from that hospital," said Dr. Green.

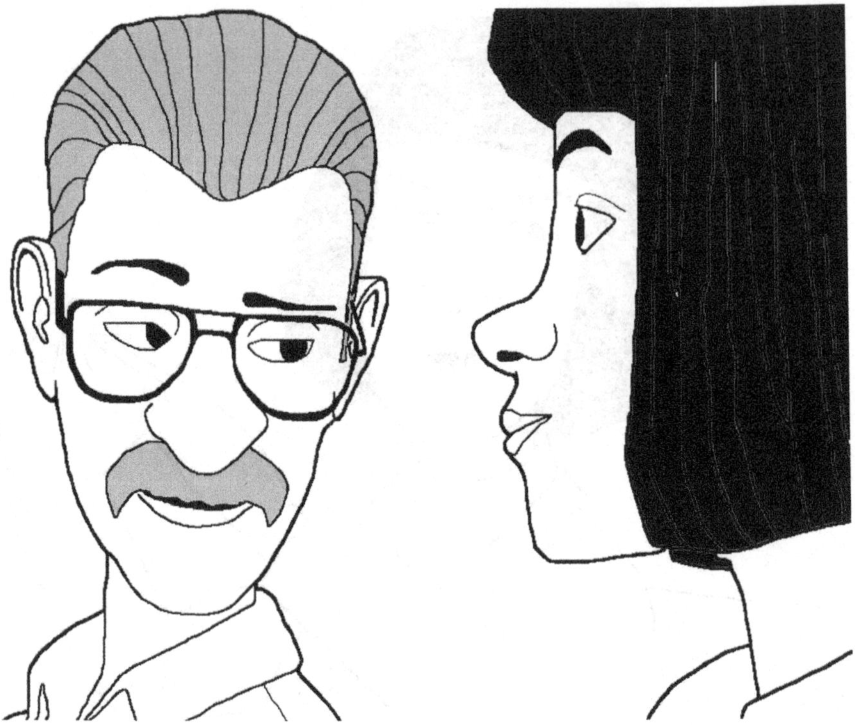

"I know I am never going back there," said Dr. Smith. "University hospital might be further away, but the extra drive is worth it in order to be treated by physicians."

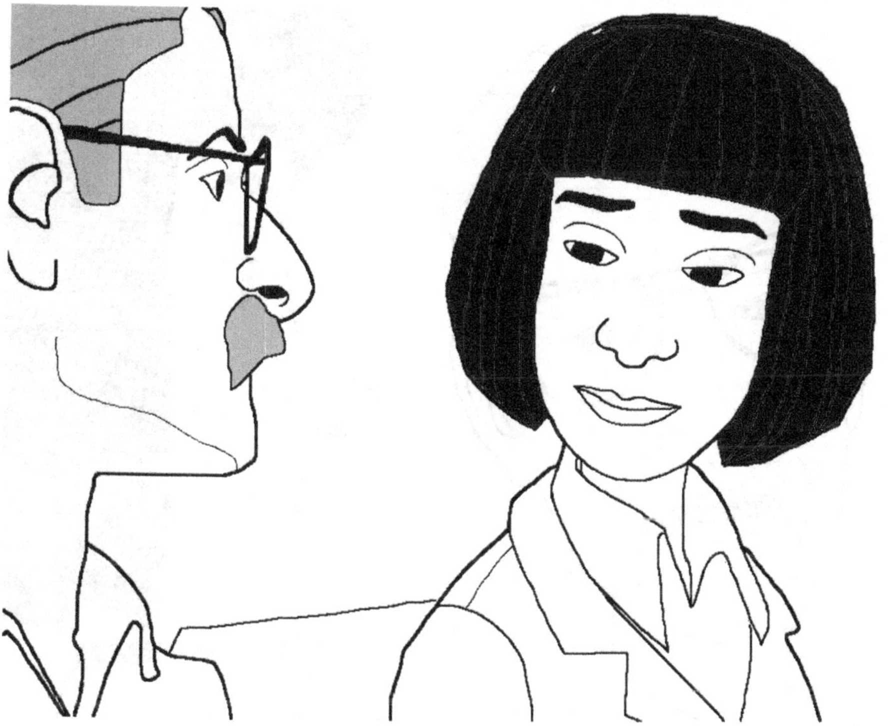

"Nurse practitioners, physician assistants, pharmacists, nurse anesthetists, physical therapists and psychologists all play important roles in a hospital," said Dr. Smith. "But a physician is the only one with thc specialized training and experience to properly diagnose and treat patients."

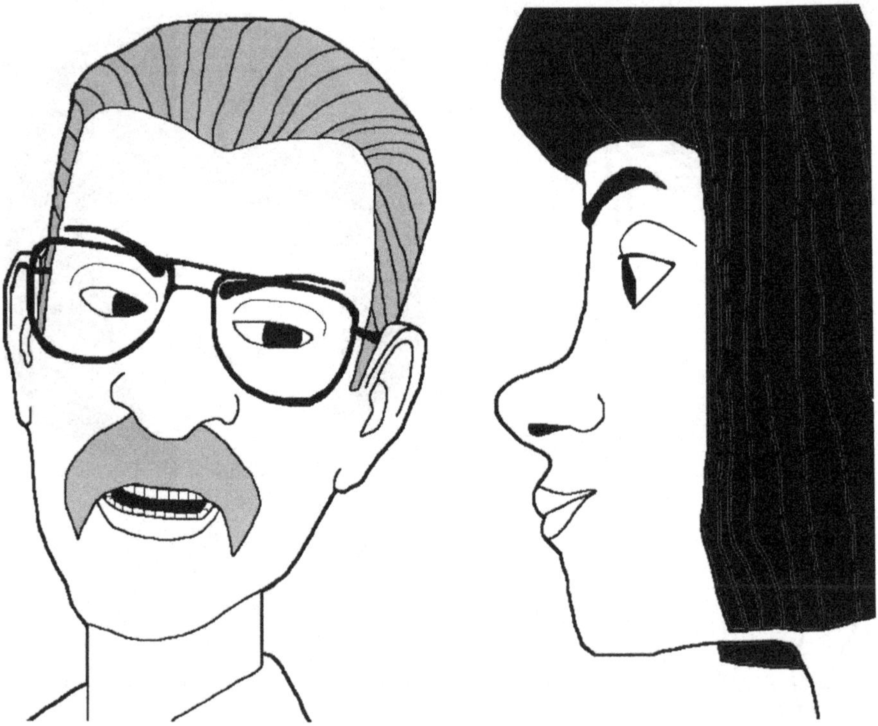

"Can you believe that in half of the country, nurse practitioners can now practice without a supervising physician?" asked Dr. Smith.

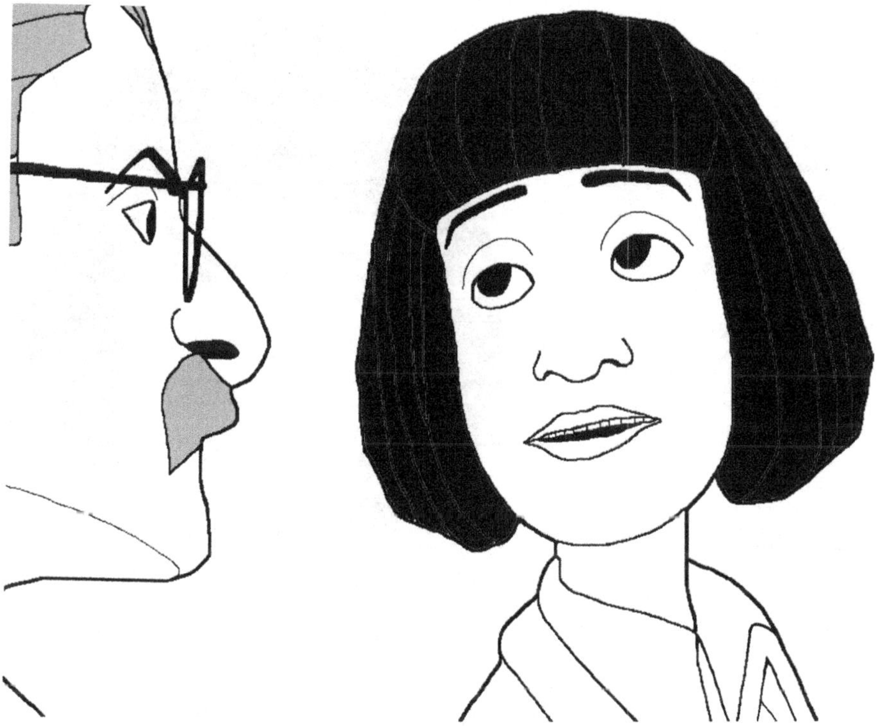

"I know," sighed Dr. Green. "I cannot believe we have become one of those states. And every year there is a push to change the laws in the other states too."

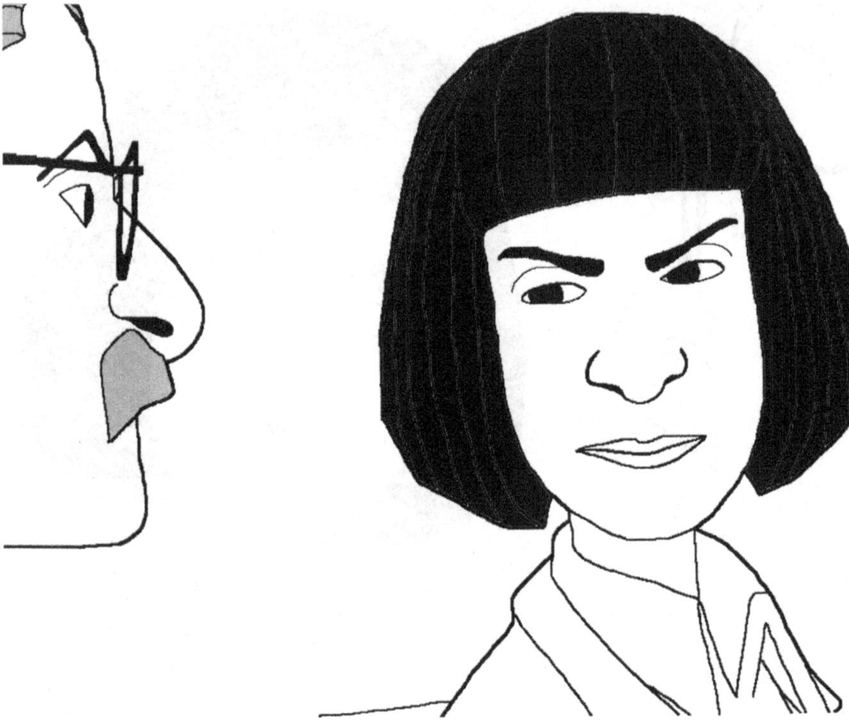

"They convince state politicians that independent practice will allow nurse practitioners to increase healthcare access in rural areas without enough primary care physicians.

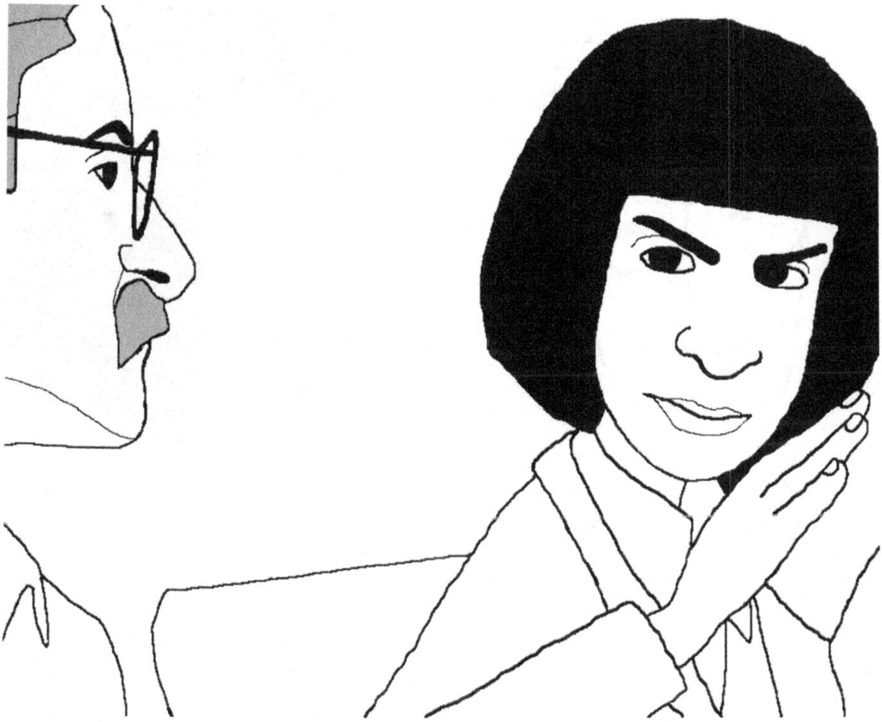

"But the data shows that they don't wind up working in rural areas," Dr. Green continued. "And many give up on the idea of doing primary care to work in cash-only medical spas, where they do cosmetic injections instead."

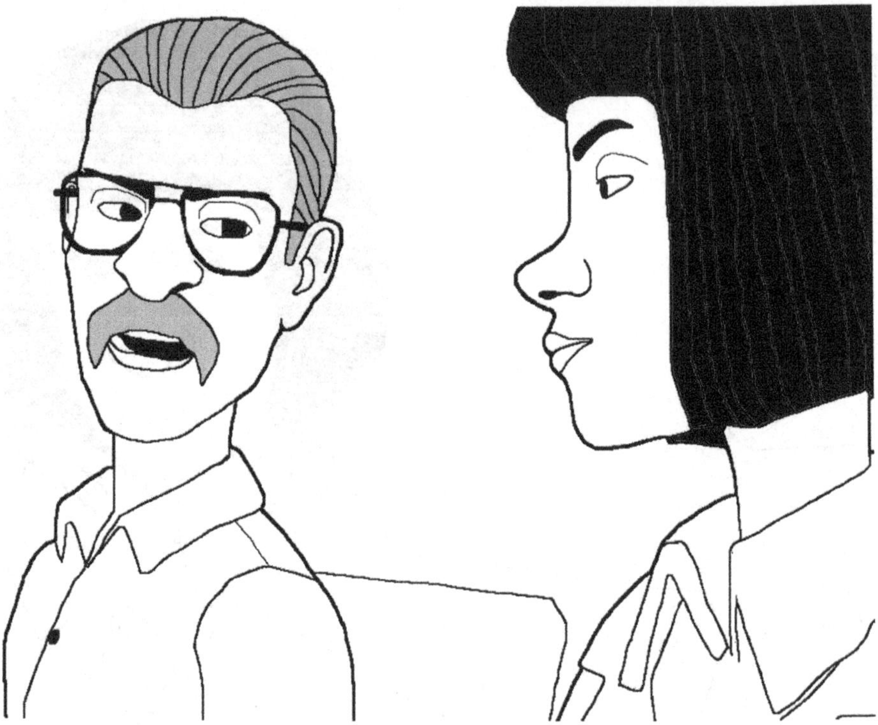

"And they are regulated by state nursing boards, not the state medical boards that oversee physicians," said Dr. Smith.

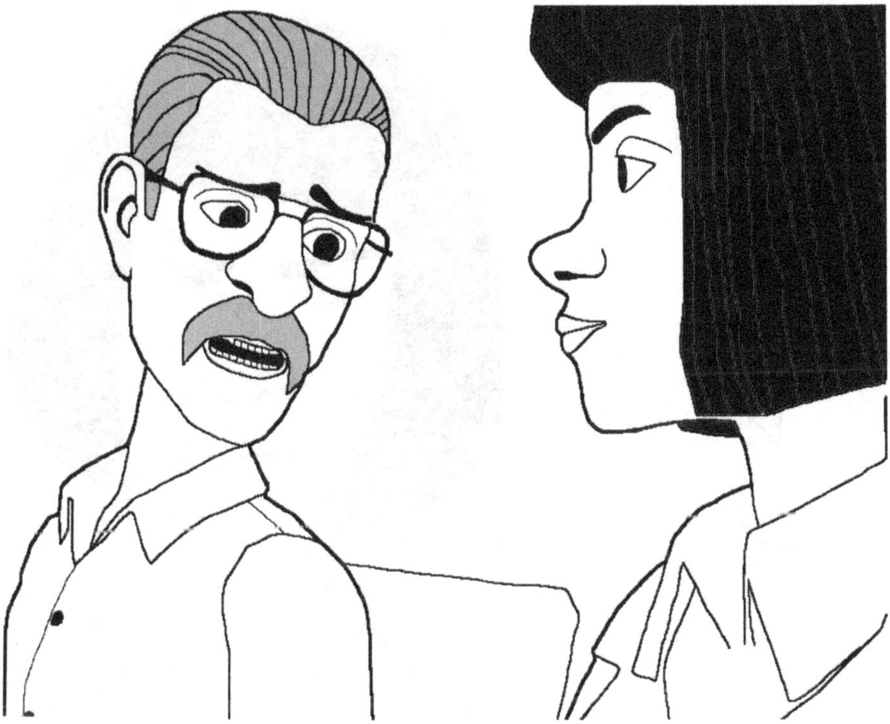

"Nurse practitioners say they are practicing advanced nursing. But diagnosing and treating patients is practicing medicine," added Dr. Smith.

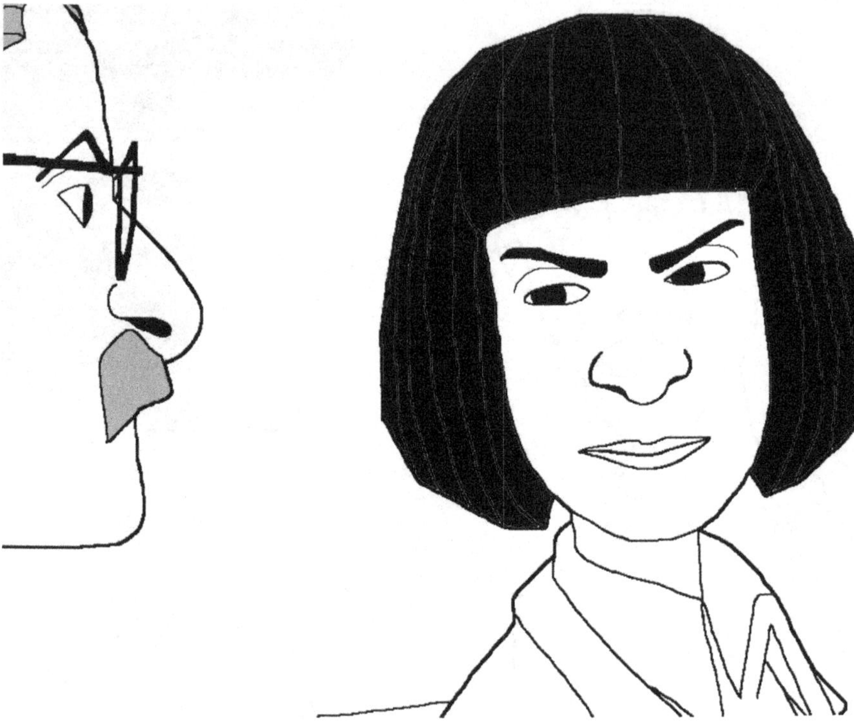

"I have heard horror stories about patients being misdiagnosed and incorrectly treated by nurse practitioners without physician supervision," agreed Dr. Green.

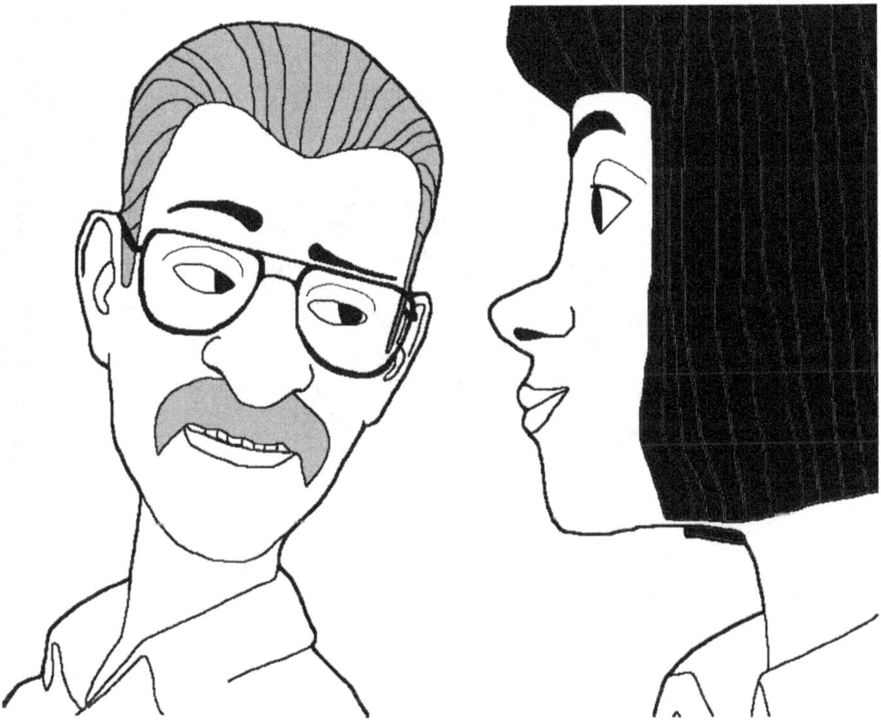

"Those nurse practitioners have powerful lobbying groups behind them," said Dr. Smith. "They got the right to practice medicine by legislation, not education."

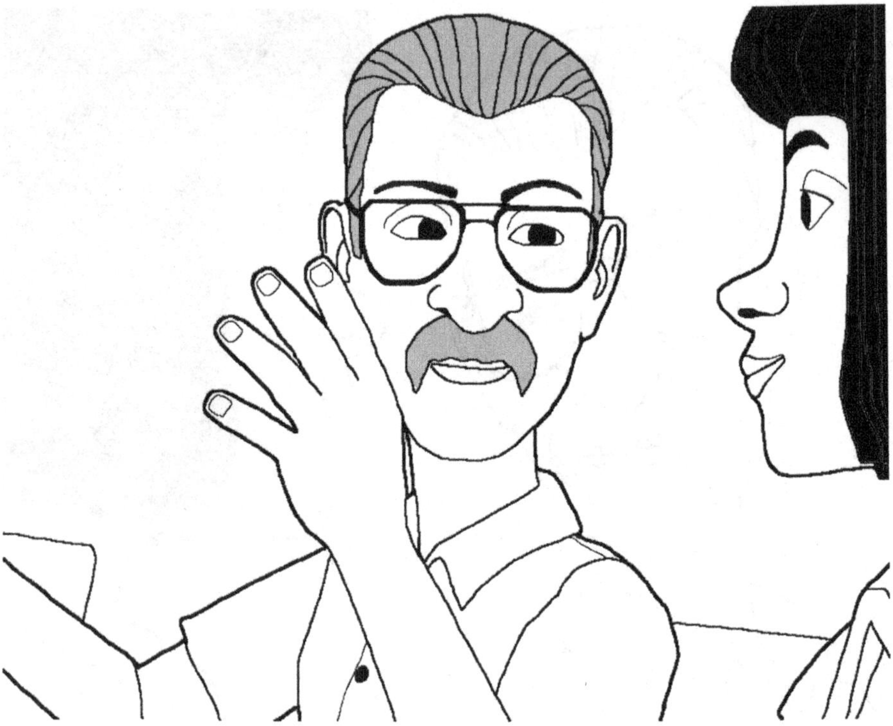

"Did you know a big pet store chain insists its dog groomers have more hands on training hours than some DNP programs require for their nurse practitioners?" asked Dr. Smith.

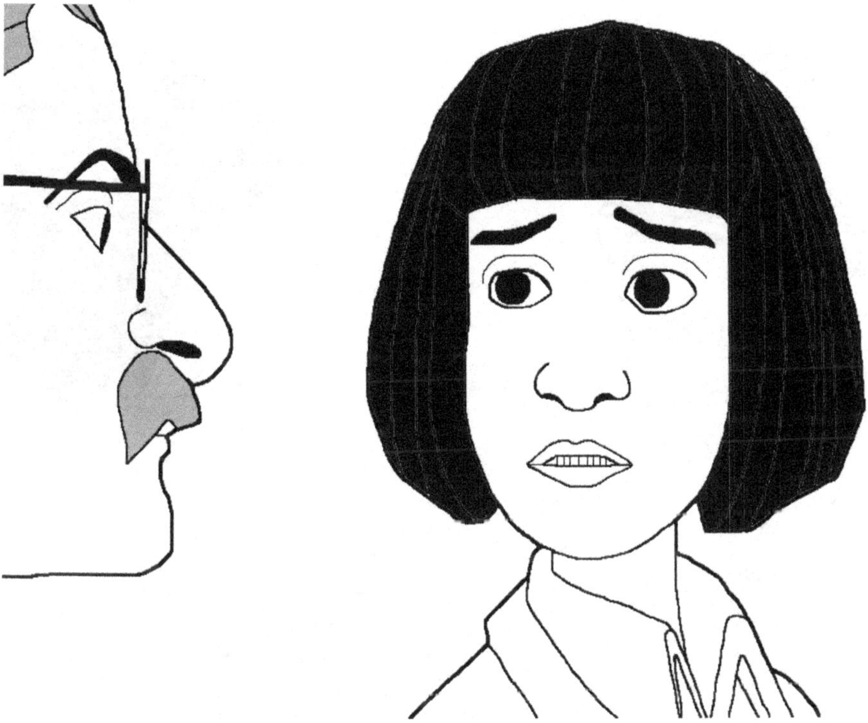

“If patients knew the truth they would not be happy,” said Dr. Green. “Please tell your friends what happened to you and tell them to ask to see the physician on their healthcare team.”

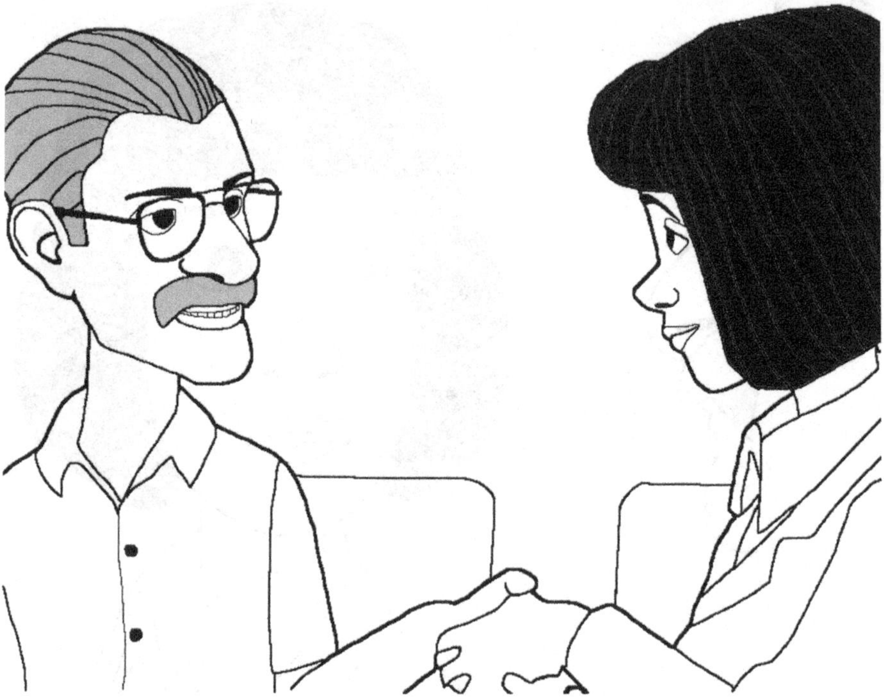

“Thank you for being my physician,” said Dr. Smith.

THE END

Made in the USA
Monee, IL
04 November 2026

67384399R00066